THE ELECTROPHYSIOLOGY OF EXTRAOCULAR MUSCLE

THE
ELECTROPHYSIOLOGY
OF EXTRAOCULAR
MUSCLE

With Special Reference to
Electromyography

By

GOODWIN M. BREININ

Published for the
American Ophthalmological Society
by University of Toronto Press
Toronto, 1962

TO ROSE-HELEN

PREFACE

It is the author's intent in this monograph to review the electrophysiology of extraocular muscle, particularly the scientific literature on ocular electromyography. Recent studies from the author's laboratory on the physiologic and pharmacologic properties of extraocular muscle are also described. The work was written as a candidate's thesis for membership in the American Ophthalmological Society.

The literature of ocular electromyography is quite recent but the bibliography is growing at a rapid rate. Fundamental advances in knowledge of extraocular muscle function in health and disease have accrued from these investigations, which are being conducted in laboratories around the world. The author has attempted to present a comprehensive summary of information on the theoretical and practical applications of electromyography to the extraocular muscles and the contributions of the technique to the general problem of strabismus.

Controversial observations are discussed at length with a critical examination of the relative merits of differing viewpoints.

Experimental studies are reported which show that extraocular muscle, contrary to the commonly accepted notion that it is primitive and unique, is actually much the same as peripheral skeletal muscle in physiologic and pharmacologic properties and in reaction to disease. The differences are found to be quantitative rather than qualitative, reflecting the highly specialized function of extraocular muscle. The author, therefore, believes in a unitary approach to the physiology and pathology of extraocular and peripheral skeletal muscle.

New bioelectronic computing techniques are reported which, through integration and differentiation, constitute a calculus of muscle innervation. An approach to electronic automation of neuromuscular diagnosis is described in myasthenia gravis. Spectrum analysis of electromyographic potentials may prove a useful aid in the differentiation of the normal from neurogenic and myogenic disorders.

Through such studies, our understanding of the innervational control of ocular motility has been placed upon a firmer footing and the relevance of mechanical-electronic servo models indicated.

The equipment and techniques employed in ocular electromyography are discussed as well as the difficulties and problems inherent in bioelectric instrumentation.

It is of interest that one of the most celebrated doctrines of neurophysiology—Sherrington's reciprocity law—was based in large part on studies of the extraocular muscles. Modern electrophysiologic techniques have provided the finest demonstration of this law. Equally basic principles are emerging from current studies. It seems reasonable to expect that continued research will add much to our fund of basic information. The practical value of electromyography to disturbances of the extraocular muscles has proved much the same as in peripheral neuromuscular disorders.

The technique has had a salutary influence in promoting joint neurologic and ophthalmologic investigation with considerable benefit to both disciplines. It has also illustrated the value of the team approach employing ophthalmologist, neurophysiologist, and electronic engineer.

Future research directed to the mechanisms of central nervous system control of muscle discharge patterns, to the role of centrally and peripherally acting drugs, to microelectrode properties and electron microscope characteristics of extraocular muscle, should lead to a profounder understanding of ocular motility control mechanisms and provide a rational physio-pathologic basis for classification of ocular motility disorders.

Deep appreciation is extended to my loyal aids in these studies: Freeman York, B.S., who ably assisted in most of the examinations and whose skill in fabrication of instruments is unique; George Thomas, E.E., who has provided engineering guidance and advice; and Walter Lentschner, invaluable and indefatigable photographer. I should also like to acknowledge with appreciation the close collaboration of James Perryman, PH.D., in the animal physiology and pharmacology studies.

I am indebted to Drs. Harris Ripps, Irwin Siegel, and Ronald Carr for their aid in editing the proofs.

I must also thank the many residents and practicing colleagues who channeled interesting patients into our many-channeled laboratory.

I wish to express my gratitude to the various sources of financial support of these studies: The National Institute of Neurological Diseases and Blindness of the United States Public Health Service, The Fight for Sight League of the National Council to Combat Blindness, and The Eye Surgery Fund.

G.M.B.

CONTENTS

THE ELECTROPHYSIOLOGY OF EXTRAOCULAR MUSCLE

with special reference to Electromyography

INTRODUCTION

INVESTIGATION OF THE STRUCTURE and function of extraocular muscle in man and lower animals has been most extensive during the past decade. The development of new electronic instrumentation and its application to bioelectric signals has permitted intensive exploration of electrophysiologic activity of nerve and muscle. This is a continuing process which promises to reveal much that is presently unknown concerning neuromuscular function. The parallel development of more delicate histologic techniques such as are provided by the electron microscope will expand knowledge of the physical substrate for much of the electrophysiologic data.

The electric activity of the eye may be divided into the corneoretinal potentials (the electroretinogram, the electro-oculogram), the autonomic muscle potentials of ciliary and iris muscles, and the electric potential of extraocular muscle (the electromyogram).

An enormous literature has accumulated about the electroretinogram and electro-oculogram, very little concerning ocular autonomic muscle potentials, while there is a steadily growing number of electromyographic studies of extraocular muscle.

In this thesis, historical and current knowledge of the electrical activity of extraocular muscle with related pharmacologic and physiologic data will be presented, including unpublished experimental observations in man and animals.

HISTORICAL SURVEY

In the nineteenth and early part of the twentieth century, the mechanical myogram of muscle contraction was recorded by many investigators. The underlying electric basis of innervation, however, required the more precise tools which were to be evolved later.

The electrophysiologic era was ushered in by Dubois-Reymond[60] who, in 1848, established the action current principle or wave of electric negativity of the nerve impulse. In 1907, Piper[116] obtained the first recorded electromyogram by means of a string galvanometer. The analysis of bioelectric potentials with the string galvanometer was necessarily limited and in 1926 the employment of the cathode-ray oscilloscope by Erlanger and Gasser[64,65] and others resulted in a giant step forward in the demonstration by the inertia-free electron beam of the electric impulse of nerve and muscle. In 1929, Adrian and Bronk[2] further implemented the analysis of electric potentials in tissues by means of the concentric needle electrode with its more limited and selective pickup.

In 1893, Sherrington [124,125] demonstrated the famous law of reciprocal innervation. In subsequent studies[126] on reciprocal innervation, he employed mechanical analysis of the contraction of antagonist extraocular muscles. In 1911, Bartels[9] recorded the mechanical nystagmogram in rabbits. Hoffmann,[70] in 1913, demonstrated action currents in rabbits' extraocular muscle with a string galvanometer, recording the tonic activity at rest and the activity during nystagmus. In 1922 and 1923, Kollner and Hoffmann[81,82] described the influence of the vestibular apparatus upon the innervation of extraocular muscle in rabbits during nystagmus and established the tetanic nature of both the fast and the slow components. They also showed the tonic activity in extraocular muscle. Their technique was improved by Perez-Cirera,[115] in 1932, who recorded the mechanical nystagmogram and electromyogram with greater fidelity. Using a mechanical "frictionless" myograph, Cooper and Eccles,[51] in 1930, investigated the mechanical and electrical responses of the internal rectus of decerebrate cats to tetanic stimulation with a neon stimulator. They showed that the response of the extraocular muscle to single and repetitive stimuli was very fast and was associated with a very brief contraction time (7.5 msec.). They demonstrated the high rate of tetanic fusion (350 cycles per sec.) and high tension (100 Gm.) produced. Muscles with longer contraction times had lower fusion frequencies. In general, however, the extraocular muscle responded in a manner comparable with peripheral skeletal muscle. Both types of muscle exhibited S-shaped tension curves in relation to frequency of stimulation.

Lorente de Nó,[94,95] in 1935, recorded action currents from extraocular muscles using both a string galvanometer and a cathode-ray oscillograph and described the features of neuromuscular conduction in these muscles. He demonstrated the time relationship between antagonists during nystagmus in rabbits with simultaneous isometric myograms and electromyograms. A maximum angular acceleration of 150° per sec. was obtained with a high frequency of synchronized twitches reaching 200 per sec. He observed an asynchronism of antagonistic muscles in nystagmus and suggested that time-delay circuits were responsible. He concluded that reciprocal innervation could not be due to a fixed anatomical mechanism since often only one muscle was active, and that the mechanism of reciprocity in nystagmus was optional. He observed, however, that cocontraction of antagonists in nystagmus occurred only after lesions of the nervous system. It also occurred in the retraction reflex of the eye.

Hoffmann,[71] in 1929, had recorded the absence of the stretch reflex in extraocular muscle. This problem was reinvestigated by McCouch and Adler[101] in 1932. Using a mechanical myograph they were unable to demonstrate stretch reflexes in extraocular muscles of decerebrate cats; hence they denied the early theory of Bartels,[10] in which proprioceptors in the extraocular muscles were held responsible for the quick component of nystagmus. De Kleyn,[53] in 1922, had also disputed the peripheral role of extraocular muscle in determining the fast component of nystagmus. Selective local anesthesia failed to alter the rhythm or character of nystagmus in rabbits; hence he maintained that nystagmus was centrally generated. During nystagmus a tension of between 10 and 20 Gm., and occasionally more than 40 Gm., was recorded.

In 1939, McIntyre[102] studied the quick component of nystagmus in the cat. He recorded action potentials in the sixth cranial nerve with an oscillograph and detected a tonic discharge of impulses which was unaffected after distal severance of the nerve. The motor impulses underlying nystagmus were characteristic. After the third, fourth, and sixth nerves had been cut bilaterally with extirpation of the retractor bulbi muscles, labyrinthine stimulation still produced characteristic nystagmus impulses in the central end of the sixth nerve. He concluded, as did McCouch and Adler, that the experiments established the truth of de Kleyn's contention that the rhythm of nystagmus was entirely central in origin and was independent of impulses from the extraocular muscles.

Duke-Elder and Duke-Elder,[61] in 1930, demonstrated by myogram and *in vitro* experiments that the extraocular muscles of the dog and cat responded to choline, acetylcholine, and nicotine with a slow tonic contraction, this being the only recorded example of such a response occurring in non-denervated adult voluntary muscle of mammals. Both intact and isolated muscles were studied. They suggested that the ocular muscles of mammals resemble the voluntary muscles of lower animals (amphibia, birds) or the voluntary muscles of mammalia before they have received their motor nerve supply or following denervation. They further suggested that this response indicated an archaic and primitive mechanism in extraocular muscle which has been lost by other voluntary muscle of mammals, and considered that a rich and anomalous nerve supply may underlie this behavior.

In 1941, Brown and Harvey[42] investigated neuromuscular transmission in the extraocular muscles of decerebrate cats with a combined electromyogram and mechanical myogram technique. They injected various drugs and also stimulated the third nerve. They pointed out that the small temporal dispersion of the twitch response in extraocular muscle makes the gross action potential nearly as useful as that of a single fiber. The small temporal dispersion was attributed to the low innervation ratio and the apparent homogeneity of physiological properties of the muscle fibers. They demonstrated the greater sensitivity to curare of extraocular muscle and suggested that this sensitivity is a reflection of the nearly identical excitability of all the fibers of such muscle. Acetylcholine produced a contraction of long duration associated with action potentials. Following eserine, however, acetylcholine and repetitive nerve stimulation evoked a contracture which blocked the propagation of excitation along the muscle fiber.

Reid,[119] in 1949, reported on the rate of discharge of extraocular motor neurones in cats and goats. Using wire electrodes he elicited a large number of high-frequency insertion potentials with rates exceeding 200 per sec. The insertion potentials also occurred while the electrodes were apparently at rest in the muscle, and were attributed to injury to motor units. Skeletal muscle does not normally reveal any electrical activity at rest, and the insertion potentials of extraocular muscle seemed more readily elicited than those of peripheral skeletal muscle. Electrical records of both nerve and muscle were obtained. Single fiber preparations of the nerve to the inferior oblique in two cats revealed no resting activity. When the head was rotated, bursts of activity occurred. Stimulation of the labyrinths with increasing intensity produced a response in the nerve to the extraocular muscles of increased frequency of individual unit discharge and recruitment of new units. Reid reported rates of discharge of muscle motor units of between 120 and 175 per sec. elicited by means of head twists. Such rates were considerably higher than any reported in peripheral skeletal muscle. Nevertheless, slow rates of discharge were common. Asynchronous discharge of motor units occurred with no evidence of rotation of activity of individual units. Such asynchronous activity was held responsible for the smoothness of tetanus. The response of denervated muscle to electrode insertion he attributed to the richness of nerve fiber supply.

Gordon,[68] in 1951, investigated the electric behavior of the lid in the baboon. He described the reciprocity in blinks between orbicularis and levator. Levator units fired at a rate of 15–50 per sec. with eyes open and were inhibited during the blink. The orbicularis reached rates of 180 per sec. at the same time. Inhibition of the levator preceded and outlasted the contraction of the orbicularis.

In 1952, Pulfrich[118] reported upon the action currents of extraocular muscles in rabbits. Using a cathode-ray oscilloscope, he clearly demonstrated the resting tonus of extraocular muscle (Ruhetonus). In nystagmus, the action currents demonstrated, in both rapid and slow phases, recruitment in frequency and amplitude of motor units in the agonist and inhibition in the antagonist. He showed the purity of reciprocal innervation in antagonistic extraocular muscles; the contraction of the agonist and relaxation of the antagonist in the fast phase occurring at the same moment. This precise reciprocity was altered by narcosis with ether and barbiturates. He further corroborated the high frequency of firing of extraocular motor units.

Bornschein and Schubert,[23] in 1952, reported upon the electromyography of rotatory nystagmus in rabbits. The action potentials of the extraocular muscles were found to be uninfluenced by isolation of the muscle from other muscles or from the globe. This held for both active and inhibitory phases. The authors found a definite relationship between the amplitude of nystagmus and the summated action potentials of the muscle.

In 1952, in a short, pioneering communication, Bjork[14] reported on the sampling of the electric activity of human extrinsic eye muscles with needle electrodes. This was the first clear-cut demonstration of extraocular muscle potentials in man, and was the prelude to a series of studies,[14–19] partly in collaboration with Kugelberg, which established human extraocular electromyography. The electric activity of the levator and recti muscles of the eye was analyzed. In comparison with peripheral skeletal muscle it was noted that the amplitude of motor units was considerably lower (between 20 and 150 μv.), the duration much shorter (between 1 and 2 msec.), and the frequency much higher (up to 150 cycles per sec.), compared with an amplitude of 100 to 3,000 μv., a duration of 5 to 10 msec., and frequencies up to

50 per sec. in the peripheral skeletal musculature. Bjork attributed
these differences to the small innervation ratio of the motor unit in
extraocular muscle. The frequency of single action potentials reached
higher levels than any known for the peripheral musculature. In strong
voluntary contractions, measurement of frequency was not possible
because the interference activity of other units obscured the picture.
Some units demonstrated an initial high frequency of 50–70 per sec.
in contrast to peripheral musculature which usually begins at a frequency below 10 per sec. and reaches a maximum of 30–50 per sec.
These rates in the human extraocular muscles compare quite closely
with those found in animals.[118-119] Bjork stated that in neurogenic
lesions of the extraocular muscles the degree of paresis could be
demonstrated electrically. Peripheral neurone disturbances showed a
considerable reduction in the number of action potentials. Fibrillations
of denervation, although difficult to distinguish from motor unit activity, could be characterized by their lower frequency, irregular
rhythm, and independence of voluntary contraction.

In 1953, Bjork and Kugelberg[15] reported on characteristics of motor
unit activity in human extraocular muscles. Observations were made
upon nineteen normal adults and upon three patients with pareses of
eye muscles. Monopolar electrodes were preferred to the concentric
because of the lesser traumatism involved. With gaze out of the field of
action, the electric activity was reduced to single unit firing. With gaze
into the field of action, the units increased in frequency of discharge
and additional units of varying amplitude were recruited. Recruitment
was more rapid than in peripheral muscle. The levator palpebrae
superioris showed a similar pattern of recruitment and frequency
increase. This had also been noted in the baboon levator.[68] In contrast
with peripheral skeletal musculature, where frequencies up to 80–90
per sec. in paretic muscles were obtained, the units of paretic extraocular muscles could rise to frequencies of 200 per sec. The form of
motor unit potentials was quite uniform and polyphasic potentials were
rarely seen, in contrast with peripheral musculature where polyphasic
potentials are not uncommon. The mean duration of the levator action
potential was reported as slightly longer than that of the recti muscles.
The mean duration of action potentials in the recti muscles was reported as 1.6 msec. with an average amplitude of 108 μv., although
units up to 500 μv. were observed. It was pointed out that the amplitude of the potential varies with the distance of the electrode from the
motor unit in question as well as other factors. The high frequency of
firing of extraocular motor units was considered related to the high
tetanic fusion frequency of eye muscles.[51] The rarity of polyphasic

potentials was attributed to the anatomic uniformity of extraocular motor units.

The fields of action of the extraocular muscles and levator palpebrae were clearly shown by Bjork and Kugelberg[16] in 1953. The levator was seen to recruit maximally in gaze upward and to become silent in extreme gaze downward. It was also silent when the eyes were closed. The orbicularis oculi had a reciprocal relationship with the levator demonstrated during blinks. The inhibition of the levator preceded and outlasted the burst of activity of the orbicularis. This had also been noted in the baboon.[68] At the extreme of movement out of the field of a muscle the electric activity was minimal or extinguished, although insertion of an electrode at different sites in some cases could bring into evidence other unit firings. The tonic firing of the extraocular muscle in the primary position was clearly demonstrated and it was noted to persist in darkness although it was obliterated during sleep. Gliding movements of the eye demonstrated a nice reciprocity mechanism between horizontal recti with gradual inhibition of the antagonist paralleling the augmentation of the agonist. By contrast, saccadic movements produced abrupt activation of the agonist with abrupt inhibition of the antagonist. At the cessation of the saccade the heightened activity of the agonist and inhibition of the antagonist disappeared rapidly with a return to that level of activity characteristic of the new position of the eye. Slight overshoots were, however, characteristic and were compensated by a rapid oscillation. The saccade duration was estimated to correspond to an angular velocity of 125° per sec. which correlated well with the values obtained by other methods. In downward movements of the eyelid there was little or no activity in the orbicularis, suggesting that downward movement was brought about mainly by relaxation of the levator. During fixation, the horizontal recti demonstrated small, synchronous potentials repeating at regular intervals. These were considered to relate to the fine, jerky movements which constantly occur during such fixation. The continuous, tonic activity was considered to stabilize movement, counteracting overshooting and oscillation during fixation. The high frequency of unit firing and persistent activity were held to subject the neuromuscular mechanism of the extraocular muscles to greater strain, and hence were a predisposing factor toward heterophoria and susceptibility to myasthenia gravis.

Glees,[67] in 1953, reported upon the electromyography of extraocular muscles in animals, employing a technique in which the muscles were held in clamps.

In 1953, Adler[1] reported upon the electromyogram of the lateral rectus in man and described an increase in the frequency and amplitude of discharge during divergence. Both in version and vergence into the field of action of the muscle there was an increase in discharge of pulses preceding the actual movement of the eye. An estimate of the frequency of firing showed no change of tonic activity in the lateral rectus in gaze straight up or straight down. He declared, therefore, that an active divergence mechanism must exist. In his studies divergence was obtained from the near point of convergence.

The electromyogram of the lateral rectus muscle in rabbits was investigated by Magee.[97] Because of inadequacy of technique the records are not clear. Nevertheless, he demonstrated the blocking effect of retrobulbar injection upon the tonic electric activity of extraocular muscle.

Bjork[17] reported on the electromyographic study of ocular palsies in 24 patients; most were due to neurogenic pareses and several to mechanical limitations of the globe. In lesions of the peripheral motor neuron, there was a reduction in the number of action potentials. The remaining potentials were similar in duration and form to the normal, but polyphasic potentials were recorded in three cases. Fibrillations, the characteristic sign of denervation, were recorded definitely in one case and probably in two others. The problem in recognizing such potentials in extraocular muscle was due to their similarity to normal potentials and because complete voluntary relaxation of eye muscle was difficult to achieve. Uneven activation of the action potentials was characteristic in a number of cases. This was associated with muscle paretic nystagmus. A tendency to grouping of potentials was also seen.

The degree of paresis could be well determined by electromyography. In most cases, clinically total palsies were shown to retain voluntary electric activity in the muscles. With severe palsies, the progress of the condition could be followed well so long as the number of potentials remained small. In moderate or mild palsies, no reduction of action potentials could be observed due to the abundance of residual motor units.

Electromyography assisted in differentiating between neuromuscular paresis and limitation of movement due to other factors since the muscles fired normally in mechanical limitations.

In a further study in 1954, Bjork[18] reported on the coordination of antagonistic muscles in abducens and facial palsy. Six patients with abducens palsy, ten with facial palsy, and five normal individuals were studied. In abducens palsy, in different positions of fixation with the good eye and during movement of gaze, the electric activity of the internal rectus, antagonist to the paretic muscle, showed a picture which would have been expected had the eye been able to assume normal positions and carry out normal movements. The activity of the antagonist to the paretic muscle diminished as the sound eye moved into the field of action of the paretic muscle and disappeared almost entirely in extreme gaze into that field. The paretic eye, however, did not achieve a direct mid-line position during this movement, indicating the presence of contracture. These alterations were independent of fixation by either the sound or the paretic eye and occurred equally well when both were covered. In nystagmus the inhibitions characteristic of the rapid phase also occurred despite the total palsy of the agonist. In facial palsy the activity of the levator muscle followed the normal pattern, becoming extinguished on extreme downward gaze. Thus, lowering of the eyelid was independent of the orbicularis muscle. Forced movements of the eye by means of bridle sutures did not alter the activity of agonist or antagonist. The electric activity corresponded always with the volitional intention of the subject as disclosed by the position of the freely moving eye.

Bjork stated that, in concomitant strabismus from infancy, a different situation is encountered. Here, the squinting eye seemed to be in muscular equilibrium when the gaze was straight ahead no matter which eye was fixing. In the squinting position the same activity was found as would be expected if a non-squinting eye assumed the same position. The above points will be discussed subsequently.

Normal human extraocular muscle electromyograms were obtained by Kuboki[84] in 1954. He analyzed the motor units as consisting of one, two, or three phases with amplitudes below 200 μv. and with a frequency of 10–70 cycles per sec. He presented a time series analysis of unit firing, describing slow and fast rhythms of discharge attributed to tonic and kinetic units respectively.

Breinin and Moldaver,[26] in 1955, reported electromyographic observations upon the normal kinesiology of extraocular muscle and described the divergence mechanism. The tonic activity of the primary position was demonstrated along with the increased frequency and recruitment which occurred as the eye rotated into the field of action of the muscle being tested. The reciprocal relationship of direct and contralateral antagonists was also clearly shown as a graded augmentation of discharge in the agonist with concomitant, graded inhibition of activity in the antagonist. Complete inactivity of electrical discharge in the extraocular muscles was not encountered except during the most extreme movements out of the field of action. The activity was not always completely inhibited, however, and low-grade single-unit firing might continue. The electric field of action of an inferior oblique was studied, which demonstrated increased firing in the upward fields, more marked nasally than temporally. Complete inhibition occurred in downward gaze. The horizontal recti maintained approximately the same level of activity in gaze up and down as in the primary position. In a patient with a complete third nerve paralysis and no volitional electric activity, fibrillation potentials were observed in the levator palpebrae and in the medial rectus. This patient subsequently rein-nervated the muscles with the electric pattern of the misdirection syndrome. The reciprocal relationship of the levator palpebrae superioris and the orbicularis oculi demonstrated by Bjork and Kugel-berg[16] was confirmed in this study and the characteristics of extraocular muscle motor units were seen to correspond closely with their description.[15]

Convergence was found to be characterized by an increase in ampli-tude, frequency, and recruitment of units in the medial recti whereas the lateral recti were progressively inhibited. On conjugate movement of the eyes to one side following a maximum convergence, a greater electric activity was produced in the agonist medial rectus. This paralleled the greater rotation of the version movement and demon-strated the active role of the medial rectus in that movement.

Patients with intermittent exotropia were studied to elucidate the nature of divergence. The lateral rectus demonstrated markedly in-creased activity at the break from the near point of convergence. This activity appeared to overlap the maximal activity of the medial rectus for some 20 msec., following which the medial rectus became inhibited. As the eye swung out in divergence, the lateral rectus activity increased and remained active. In another patient with intermittent exotropia, the lateral rectus of the diverging eye demonstrated a marked increase of firing on breaking from fusion into exotropia with remote fixation. An attempt to determine fusional divergence activity with prisms was not successful because of the limited amplitude of divergence. These observations conclusively established the active nature of divergence and rendered untenable the passive concept of divergence as due solely to inhibition of the medial rectus with divergence stress pro-duced by mechanical factors. The source of such active divergence innervation, however, remained unknown.

The consistency in reproducibility of electromyographic patterns despite the fact that changes of needle position must have occurred in movement was striking. A unit fired steadily in one eye position for an hour. Despite movement of the eye into other fields, on return to the same position the identical activity of the unit was obtained, suggesting a fixity of electrode-unit relationship. Forced fixation of the globe during attempted gaze movement demonstrated that the innervational pattern corresponded to that of the willed movement in a freely rotating globe. Passive movement of the globe did not alter activity, which always accorded with the volitional effort. Covering the eyes made no difference. This confirmed Bjork's description[18] of the phenomenon and indicated that the effort of innervation determined the electric activity. Electromyograms of nystagmus were described in which a fine reciprocity mechanism existed between antagonistic muscles. Extremely rapid rates of nystagmus could be displayed in detail by the electromyographic technique.

In 1955, Breinin[27] reported on the nature of vergence revealed by electromyography. He cited the finding that in intermittent exotropia the deviating eye showed an appropriate alteration of its horizontal recti, but that no change was apparent in the muscles of the fixing eye. In short, only the moving eye exhibited an alteration of innervation. Experimentally, in asymmetric convergence the deviating eye showed large alterations of innervation with increased activity of the medial rectus and inhibition of the lateral rectus. The non-moving eye, on the other hand, showed little or no change of innervation. A simple scheme was presented to show the algebraic summation of innervation of version and vergence in the heterotropias and in asymmetric vergence. Heterotropia and asymmetric convergence could be analyzed, therefore, in terms of a dual movement of vergence and version which, in the case of the moving eye, created addition of innervation in the agonist and inhibition in the antagonist. In the fixing eye, the innervations of version and vergence were of opposite sign resulting in no change in the level of innervation which previously existed; thus, no movement occurred. In the deviating eye, the additive innervations of version and vergence resulted in its greater excursion. These innervations appeared to be centrally adjusted since there was no evidence of cocontraction of antagonists in the non-moving eye. This illustrated the truth of Hering's explanation[69] of asymmetric vergence, although he placed the site of adjustment peripherally rather than centrally. This indicated that the heterotropic deviations of the eye were not simple but complex, manifesting the dual innervations of version and vergence. The importance of sensory control in policing motor disturbances was stressed. In addition, the truth of Hering's law of distributed innervation was demonstrated by electromyography.

Sakatani,[120] in 1955, reported on normal and abnormal electromyograms and described slow and fast rhythms in human extraocular muscle, also attributing these rhythms to the activity of tonic and kinetic units respectively. The Japanese investigators—Kuboki,[84-90] Kamouchi,[79-80] and Sakatani[120-121]—have gone in extensively for analyses of single motor unit frequencies, periodicities, and rhythms in extraocular muscle.

In 1955, Bjork[19] reported upon the electromyogram of the extraocular muscles in opticokinetic nystagmus and in reading. Fifty patients with normal eye movements and 15 patients with disturbed motility due to ocular paresis were studied. The levator was studied in three patients in whom the eye had been enucleated. In most of the patients the electro-oculogram, which records eye movement, was simultaneously obtained with the electromyogram. An opticokinetic drum was used for nystagmus. Both vertical and horizontal nystagmus were induced and antagonistic muscles recorded simultaneously. In both horizontal and vertical opticokinetic nystagmus, the muscles which by their contraction produced the slow phase showed continually increasing electric activity with simultaneously decreasing activity in the antagonist. In the muscles which produced the fast phase, a burst of strong activity was seen, and in the opposing muscles, as a rule, complete inhibition. The two phases of nystagmus were clearly seen in the electromyogram with a sharply marked reciprocal action between agonist and antagonist. During reading, the movements of the eyes were very similar to the opticokinetic nystagmus. During fixation pauses, the activity resembled that obtained when the eye fixates a stationary point. During slow movements of gaze without a fixation point, short jerks occurred with strong bursts of activity in the agonist and abrupt inhibition of activity in the antagonist. A similar pattern was also seen in rapid movements of gaze between two fixation points.

In 1955, Kamouchi[78] reported upon the electromyography of palsied extraocular and levator muscles, describing the characteristic change in 56 cases of oculomotor, trochlear, and abducens palsies. In general, there was a decrease in the number of normal spike discharges while abnormal discharges consisting of low-amplitude normal motor unit voltage, complex normal motor unit voltage, reinnervation voltage, and grouping voltage were demonstrated. Fibrillation voltage was not recognized.

In 1955 and 1956, Kuboki[85-86] reported upon human extraocular electromyography in a series of papers and compared extraocular with peripheral muscle electromyograms. He presented further time series (correlogram) analyses of unit discharges and described slow and fast rhythms. He reported the behavior of individual units of the horizontal recti during slow movements and found that each unit had a definite range of action; some fired independently of movement.

Huber and Lehner,[74] in 1956, reported upon ocular electromyography in normal and abnormal muscles and pointed out the importance of this technique in the diagnosis of motility disturbances. The neurogenic and myasthenic patterns were briefly described, the latter being characterized as a myopathy.

In 1956, Magee[98] described the electromyogram of the lateral rectus muscle in man. The poor quality of the recordings makes it almost impossible to evaluate the data. In one figure, however, he did show the alterations of the lateral rectus with position of gaze.

In 1957, in a series of papers, Breinin[28-35] reported on the following subjects:

1. Position of rest during anesthesia and sleep.[33]
2. The electromyographic evidence for ocular muscle proprioception in man.[30]
3. Electromyography as a tool in ocular and neurologic diagnosis of (a) myasthenia gravis[28] and (b) muscle palsies.[29]
4. Quantitation of extraocular muscle innervation.[31]
5. New aspects of ophthalmoneurologic diagnosis.[34]
6. The nature of vergence revealed by electromyography; accommodative and fusional vergence.[35]
7. Electrophysiologic insight in ocular motility.[32]
8. The effects of succinylcholine on the extraocular muscles[91] (with Lincoff and De Voe).

These papers will be discussed subsequently.

In his Montgomery lecture for 1957, Walsh[139] presented an account of third nerve regeneration in which electromyographic material demonstrating the misdirection phenomenon and other nerve lesions was discussed. A number of the electromyograms were provided by Breinin.

Huber,[75] in 1957, reported upon myasthenia gravis and the important diagnostic role of ocular electromyography. He characterized the electromyographic picture of myasthenia in the levator, orbicularis, and recti muscles as characteristic of myopathy with an increased number of potentials of short duration, small amplitude, and polyphasic nature. Histologic study of an inferior rectus revealed the characteristic changes of myopathy. The restorative effect of intravenous edrophonium chloride (Tensilon) upon the myasthenic muscle was clearly pictured. Where the myasthenic atrophy appeared irreversible, surgery was employed to correct deviations.

Blodi and Van Allen,[21] in 1957, reported upon the electric phenomena at the breakpoint of fusion in the extraocular muscles. On exceeding the near point of convergence the electric activity of the external rectus increased suddenly, while the potentials of the internal rectus decreased. This occurred regardless of the means by which convergence was elicited, that is, by haploscope, prisms, or near vision.

No change in the electric potentials of the horizontal muscles was elicited during asymmetric convergence when the tested eye did not move, confirming the observation of Breinin.[27] The breakpoint of divergence did not produce any change in the electric activity of the muscles being tested under the conditions of their experiment. They presented the theory that the sum total of innervation to the two horizontal muscles has to remain the same regardless of the position of the eye, and that any change in one horizontal rectus is paralleled by a reciprocal alteration in the other. Against this is the observation of augmenting activity in an agonist while the antagonist is either fully inhibited or maintains an invariable activity.

Kamouchi,[79] in 1956, reported on the time series analysis of discharge intervals of single motor units in the extraocular and levator palpebrae muscles. Using the technique of Nomura, a highly complex mathematical and statistical analysis of the discharge intervals of single units, he was able to confirm the existence of two types of normal motor units: one, the kinetic; the other, the tonic spike. This point of view had already been expressed by Kuboki[84] and Sakatani.[120] The former stated that the ocular muscles are considered to be more cortical than spinal in character. A rather small number of units was employed for these analyses, and in view of alterations in the signal produced by technique and apparatus, the validity of their findings remains to be established. Kamouchi reported slow and irregular undulations of discharge rhythm.

In a study on the influence of flicker stimulation on the discharge intervals of single units, Kamouchi[80] found that a few seconds after onset of flicker, spasm-like activations were observed in the interval diagrams. The slow undulation decreased and almost disappeared; irregular fluctuations also decreased. He attributed these phenomena to reflex muscle spasm due to central excitement induced by flicker stimulation and suggested that these reactions looked like arousal reactions rather than the flicker potentials obtained in electrocorticograms.

In 1957, Kuboki[87-88] reported two studies on the discharge intervals of single motor units in the human extraocular muscles. The first part concerned fixation of the gaze; the second part, movement of the eye. Fifteen normal individuals were examined. During fixation of the gaze upon a point, the discharge frequency of single units was constant, but if the gaze moved to another point it varied with the degree of contraction of the muscle studied. When the average rate of discharge was over 30 per sec., the variation of discharge interval was small and the patterns of interval diagrams uniform. When the average rate of discharge fell below 30 per sec., the variations of discharge interval increased and the pattern of diagrams also became variable. When the average rate of discharge was below 10 per sec., there was very little regularity of the discharge. The variety of discharge interval diagrams was attributed to a very complicated, rich supply of nerve fibers to the motor unit, with a consequent complicated function.

In the study of horizontal movements of the eye, discharge intervals of the single unit in the agonist decreased as a rule, while those of the antagonist increased, but a great deal of individual variation occurred. Strikingly, some units were found to discharge with constant and high frequencies regardless of the movement of the eye. Each unit of the internal and external rectus muscles had its own range of action fixed to the movement of the eye. Differences between impulsive and gliding movements were not always apparent in the behavior of each unit. In the most extreme movements of the eye out of the field of the muscle, the activity of the antagonistic muscle never fell to zero. Sometimes a few units in the antagonistic muscle were observed to increase their rate of discharge in this movement out of the field of action. He pointed out that certain units, therefore, did not obey the law of reciprocal innervation. The increase in firing of some units away from their field of action he attributed to reflex fixation or stretch reflex. Differences in single unit behavior between gliding and impulsive movements were not apparent. The smoothness of eye movement, therefore, was attributed to uniformity of discharge intervals and asynchronism of discharge of each unit with gradual recruitment or diminution of units in activity.

Kuboki *et al.*[89] reported in 1958 on the periodicity in the electromyograph of human extraocular muscles. They applied Fourier analysis to the motor units obtained with a fast sweep speed and determined that the maxima of amplitude distribution occurred in the region around 100 cycles per sec. for the primary position and 150–200 cycles per sec. in the extremely adducted position.

In a second report on the periodicity in the electromyograph of human extraocular muscles, Kuboki and associates[90] studied the internal rectus muscle in horizontal positions of the eye. In this technique it was found that periodic waves could be best obtained by not inserting the electrode, which was monopolar, directly into the muscle belly but rather removing it for some distance from the muscle. In this way it behaved somewhat as a surface electrode. This study was inspired by the original report of Piper[117] on the elucidation of the Piper rhythm in skeletal muscle, employing surface electrodes. The periodic vibrations resembling Piper rhythm were not always observed in the extraocular muscles since they varied with needle position and also the individual subject. A slow and a fast rhythm were elicited. The mode value of frequency of slow rhythm in the primary position was between 70 and 100 cycles per sec., whereas for fast rhythm occurring in the extremely adducted position it was between 150 and 250 cycles per sec. These values closely approached the maximum frequency of discharge of single units in the corresponding positions of the eye (70 cycles per sec. in the primary position and 200 cycles per sec. in the extremely adducted position).

The authors assumed that the slow and fast rhythms represented the activities of tonic and kinetic units respectively. Slow rhythm appeared in the region from about 30° abducted to the extremely adducted position of the eye. Fast rhythm appeared only at adducted positions over 30°, being superimposed on the slow rhythm.

It must be noted that analyses such as these must suffer from the extreme variability in the signal due to uncontrollable variations of technique and instrumentation. The validity of the method, observations, and conclusions remains to be determined.

Momosse[109] in 1957, studied the action of the extraocular muscles in monocular movements by means of quantification of the integrated electromyogram. Ten normal volunteers were examined and the horizontal and vertical muscles studied in secondary and tertiary positions of gaze. During asymmetric convergence the integrated electromyogram showed that no change occurred in the horizontal recti of the stationary eye. This was true in both primary and secondary directions of gaze confirming the previous observations of Breinin.[27] In consequence of this finding, he stated the theory that the quantity of innervation to each extraocular muscle is a function of the position of gaze and the moving velocity of the fixation line; when the fixation line is in repose it is a function of the position of the eye alone. In horizontal gaze, the action potentials of the agonist increased steadily with a marked increase past the zero degree point. The integrated electromyogram formed a concave curve reaching a peak at the limit of the field of fixation, the so-called shortening curve. The action potentials no longer increased despite the effort to continue rotation, but rather decreased at this extreme point. In the reverse movement away from the field of action, the integrated electromyogram curve descended gradually and at the outer limit of the field of fixation the quantity of action potentials was approximately zero. This was the so-called lengthening curve. In gliding movements of the eye he found a certain number of discharge bursts which ordinarily are encountered in impulsive movement.

The shortening and lengthening curves were generally symmetrical in shape; however, the lengthening curve quantitatively was lower than the shortening curve, indicating greater electric activity of contracting muscle over that of relaxing muscle. With increase in the velocity of shortening, the concavity of the shortening curve lessened, that is, became more nearly a linear function. However, little change occurred in the concavity of the lengthening curve with different speeds of relaxation.

In vertical movements through the primary position and horizontal secondary positions (23° in and out), the horizontal recti revealed no increase or decrease of their electric activity. In horizontal movements through the vertical secondary position (23° up and down), the electric activity was almost identical with that in the primary horizontal movement. Momosse considered that when the velocity of movement was zero the height of the integrated electromyogram curve in the vertical secondary positions was roughly equal to that of an equivalent point on the primary horizontal plane. In oblique movements the curve of the horizontal muscles was closely similar to that obtained in horizontal movements for equivalent points, with some difference in height between the two curves.

Curves of the vertical recti through the primary vertical and secondary horizontal (23° in and out) positions were similar. In horizontal movements through the primary horizontal plane and vertical secondary position (23° up and down), there was no change in electric activity. Similarity was also obtained in oblique movements, comparing corresponding points on the vertical plane. Momosse pointed out that the vertical recti and obliques cannot act as active accessory ductors of the eye, since their innervation does not alter in horizontal movements, confirming the findings of Breinin.[31]

Ambrosio, Barone, and Serra[6] reported their initial observations upon the electric activity of the extraocular muscles during intermittent light stimulation, in 1957. They elicited spikes in the internal rectus muscle corresponding to the frequency of stimulation of the strobe light without appreciable movement of the globe. No electric activity was recorded in the antagonist and in several figures there is no recordable electric activity of extraocular muscles while gazing at infinity or straight ahead. This suggests that the technique was inadequate. They hypothesized that the light pathway traverses the diencephalic region returning to the spindles of the extraocular muscles and to the ocular muscle fibers themselves.

Serra and Barone,[123] in 1957, reported initial studies on the exploration of electric activity of the extraocular muscles during the perception of form. Diverse figures and forms were submitted for inspection to five subjects. Ocular electromyograms were taken both during the inspection and subsequently when the subjects were requested to mentally recall the images they had seen. The authors described various types of electromyographic activity during the inspection and subsequent recall. They reported that the innervation of the muscles during the recall of figures resembled that seen during actual inspection of the figures, indicating that visual memory produced an outflow of innervation to the muscles. Between inspection and recall there was electric silence of the muscles.

Ambrosio and D'Esposito[7] reported on the Turk-Duane syndrome. Electromyography was carried out in six patients. The analysis of single motor units showed for the most part involvement of both internal and external rectus muscles. The average amplitude of units ranged from 30 to 40 μv. in the medial and lateral recti, whereas in the superior rectus it averaged 80 to 100 μv.

Electromyography was carried out in only four of these six patients. The clinical description of a number of these does not accord with the accepted description of the Duane syndrome. Furthermore, the technique appeared inadequate, since motility was reported as being normal in the direction of gaze of muscles which showed no electric activity or very abnormal activity in cases one to four.

In 1957, Bjork, Halldin, and Wahlin[20] reported on the enophthalmos elicited by succinylcholine and the effect of succinylcholine and noradrenaline on the intraorbital muscles in man and experimental animals. They noted a rapid onset of enophthalmos produced by succinylcholine. Electromyography was performed on 15 humans to whom succinylcholine was administered in 50-mg. doses. Enophthalmos developed within 20 seconds and lasted four to five minutes. These patients had been in the third plane of anesthesia in which electric activity disappears in the extraocular muscles. After the drug was administered, electric activity was evoked consisting of a few potentials of low amplitude and frequency lasting one-half to one minute following which electric silence developed. They saw some fine twitches in muscles which had been exposed at surgery. Contraction of the extraocular muscles was ruled out as a cause of the enophthalmos since the low activity evoked was considered too weak to be responsible for movement of the globe. They also could observe no movement of the muscle. Electric silence following the evoked activity indicated that the muscles were not operative. They noted the possibility of a non-electric contracture developing in the extraocular muscles but considered it not probable and ruled it out. They noticed in studies on animals that noradrenaline had an opposite effect to succinylcholine on the nictitating membrane of the cat. Enophthalmos was also produced by this drug in rats. Their conclusion was that the enophthalmos-producing mechanism of succinylcholine is accomplished through its action upon the smooth muscle of the orbit and not via extraocular muscle.

The experimental studies of Lincoff and associates[91-92] and of Dillon *et al.*[57] indicated that non-electric contracture of extraocular muscle is the mechanism whereby succinylcholine is capable of causing retraction of the globe with consequent elevation of intraocular pressure. The definitive proof of this has been established by strain gauge studies of the extraocular muscles in man and animals combined with electromyography.[40,41] Further observations on this problem will be presented below.

In 1957, Papst, Esslen, and Mertens[111] reported upon their clinical experiences with electromyography in ocular myopathy. They compared the normal electromyogram with that obtained in two cases of myopathy. The first was a degenerative disease consisting of slowly progressive paralysis of the external ocular muscles. The clinical picture corresponded to the so-called progressive nuclear ophthalmoplegia. Electromyography of the horizontal recti showed that although the eye muscles were almost completely paralyzed there was a profuse discharge of action potentials elicited on version effort. The defect could not be attributed to a neurogenic palsy since for such a severe degree of paresis there should have been marked loss of potentials and signs of denervation. Several other cases were examined electromyographically and histologically and proved to be muscular dystrophy.

Another type of myopathy, the inflammatory myositis, was described. This patient had no external signs of inflammation but showed multiple extraocular muscle weakness. The onset was sudden with diplopia, orbital and frontal pains. The sedimentation rate was slightly elevated. Curare and prostigmine tests were negative.

Electromyography of the horizontal recti showed an abundance of motor units whose number was in sharp contrast to the degree of palsy. There were no signs of denervation. The patient was treated with steroids with prompt regression of the ocular muscle palsies within a few days. The authors pointed out that myositis need not be accompanied by external signs of inflammation and that such cases are not at all rare, but are usually misdiagnosed as neurologic problems. They suggested that in multiple ocular muscle palsies the degenerative or inflammatory forms of myopathy should be considered. The electromyograms showed abundant interference activity with good amplitude, although the potentials were not individually analyzed.

In a report on ocular myopathies, Esslen, Mertens, and Papst[66] described a case of external ophthalmoplegia which was studied by electromyography and by histologic examination of biopsied muscle. These proved that the ophthalmoplegia was, in fact, a form of muscular dystrophy.

In a second report on chronic ocular myositis by Mertens, Esslen, and Papst,[104] four cases were discussed. These patients usually exhibited monocular exophthalmos, edema of the lids, chemosis, and multiple muscle palsies. Intraorbital tumors were usually suspected and had to be ruled out. Endocrine exophthalmos also had to be ruled out by metabolic studies. The differential diagnosis was made by histologic examination of biopsied ocular muscle and electromyography.

A third report by Mertens, Esslen, and Papst[105] described the oligo-symptomatic type of myositis in which electromyography permitted the establishment of the diagnosis. This type is described further in a subsequent paper.

The cases described in the second report were included in another publication on chronic ocular myositis by Papst, Mertens, and Esslen in 1958.[113] All seven cases presented the features of exophthalmic ophthalmoplegia. There was unilateral exophthalmos associated with lid edema, multiple ocular palsies, and transient conjunctival irritation and photophobia. In three cases, amaurosis due to simple atrophy of the optic nerve occurred during the acute stage of the disease. This complicated the diagnosis since inflammatory changes of the muscles were not thought to involve the optic nerve. Retinal folds in the absence of orbital tumors also occurred. Endocrine ophthalmopathy must always be differentiated. In myositis, lid retraction was never present, whereas ptosis was constantly present. Some inflammatory pseudotumors of the orbit were attributed to this form of ocular myositis. An impressive improvement under steroid therapy supported the interpretation of the picture as a chronic myositis of possibly rheumatic-allergic origin. Histologic examination confirmed this opinion.

Chronic ocular myositis must be differentiated from orbital tumor principally by means of electromyography, according to these investigators. Electromyography of extraocular muscles was carried out in three of the seven patients and was the decisive diagnostic adjuvant. All showed an abundance of potentials which were quickly recruited into an interference pattern in strong contrast to the extreme degree of paresis exhibited by the muscles. Furthermore, the potentials were generally of short duration, about 1 msec. No spontaneous potentials, such as fibrillation, were encountered.

Of interest was their finding of amplitudes up to 1,000 μv. Preponderantly, however, the amplitudes of units were below 100 μv. Only a few sporadic, polyphasic potentials were encountered. Of importance is the fact that such abundant activity of large-amplitude potentials was encountered in the presence of a severe clinical palsy. Of great interest was the remarkable responsiveness of these patients to corticosteroid therapy.

In a study of ocular muscle dystrophy, the so-called progressive ophthalmoplegia externa, Papst, Esslen, and Mertens[112] described the electromyographic findings in three patients. The potentials varied in amplitude from low normal to high normal, with durations of about 1.5 msec. The number of potentials was usually abundant, but in one case was greatly reduced. The most noteworthy electromyographic sign of myopathy was the fullness of action potentials in contrast to the high degree of paresis of ocular muscles. The absence of denervation potentials was notable. The authors stated that a positive diagnosis by electromyography alone was not possible. Muscle biopsies of extraocular and peripheral skeletal musculature corroborated the diagnosis of a myopathy. These authors suggested that electromyography of peripheral skeletal musculature may reveal the signs of myopathy, even in the absence of clinical weakness. The abundance of potentials was attributed to an increased firing rate in the weakened units, compensating for the paresis. They further concluded that progressive external ophthalmoplegia is not due to destruction of ganglion cells but is a special form of chronic, progressive muscular dystrophy.

Papst, Mertens, and Esslen[114] continued their study of ocular myopathies with a report on the so-called oligosymptomatic ocular myositis in 1959. They reported ten cases of varying ocular muscle paralysis verified as myopathy. Oligosymptomatic myositis was compared with exophthalmic myositis. These conditions are similar and tend to spontaneous remission and exacerbation. In the oligosymptomatic form, conjunctival inflammation is less frequent and exophthalmos does not occur. They stated that electromyography makes it possible to differentiate neurogenic paresis, ocular myasthenia, endocrine ophthalmopathy, and ocular muscular dystrophy. The patients responded quickly to corticosteroid therapy and the authors concluded that oligosymptomatic myositis belongs to the rheumatic group of collagen diseases.

It is doubtful whether advanced cases of dysthyroid ophthalmoplegia could be distinguished from the exophthalmic myositis described by these authors. Metabolic studies are not necessarily definitive. The therapeutic response to corticosteroids cited by them might constitute a therapeutic test.

In 1958, Breinin[36] reported upon supranuclear mechanisms in a continuing study of electromyography. He also described analytic studies[37] of the electromyogram of human extraocular muscles in 1958. A paper on quantitative electronic techniques in ocular motility and the Holmes lecture on contributions of electromyography to strabismus[39] were published in 1959. These will be discussed subsequently.

Momosse,[110] in 1959, reported electromyographic studies on the mechanism of limitation of monocular movement. Using the integrated electromyogram, he found that the peak horizontal limit of the horizontal rotator was higher than its oblique peak. A similar curve was obtained for vertical movers. He attributed these differences to inhibition since on extreme movement effort there resulted a decrease of potentials. From the flattening curve of the horizontal rotator 20 to 30° out of its field, he deduced an isometric element, since the absence of potentials in the antagonist meant that elastic tension was increasing up to the limit of the monocular field of fixation. The decrease of potentials beyond this point in the agonist he attributed to inhibition or exhaustion of the nucleus. The lower level of potentials in the superior rectus, inferior oblique, and lateral rectus in oblique gaze he attributed to combined inhibition.

Miller,[106] in 1958, investigated the electromyographic pattern of saccadic eye movements. The saccadic movement was exemplified by conjugate gaze shifts, while tonic movement was represented by vergence, the former having a rapid and the latter a very slow acceleration. This difference has been attributed to a dual innervation to the ocular muscles with large myelinated fibers (somatic) subserving the saccadic movement and small non-myelinated fibers (autonomic) subserving the vergence movement.[4] Concentric electrodes and a special bipolar electrode containing two very fine wires within the bore of the needle were employed. The latter was used to elicit single motor units. Miller determined that a saccadic movement was induced by a sudden burst of motor unit activity which was immediately followed by an orderly firing pattern. The duration of the initial burst was proportional to the extent of movement. Large movements were usually inadequate, requiring correction by a second saccadic burst. He stated that the rate of firing of a motor unit was related to the degree of contraction, a greater contraction bringing into play additional motor units which increased their firing frequency according to the degree of fixation away from the primary position. Motor units always fired at an orderly rate. Saccadic movements were not characterized by a checking action of the antagonist of the muscle that initiated the movement. In contrast to saccadic movement, the onset of convergence was more gradual, tending to rise to an innervational peak followed by a slow decline to the final innervational pattern.

In 1958, Tamler, Jampolsky, and Marg[129] reported an electromyographic study of asymmetric convergence. They determined that the apparent lack of movement of the stationary eye in asymmetric convergence was associated with a simultaneous increase of electric activity in both the medial and lateral rectus muscles. They stated that this agreed with Hering's theoretical prediction of a peripheral balancing of opposing vergence and version stimuli to the stationary eye. They further described a small, rapid, initial movement of the stationary eye in asymmetric convergence which agreed with the work of others employing non-electromyographic techniques. They stated that there was a peripheral manifestation of vergence and version in the horizontal recti of the stationary, fixing eye as determined by two stimulus methods: (a) smooth binocular convergence along the axis of one eye; (b) refusion movement which occurs when uncovering a previously covered abducted eye of an intermittent exotrope. They believed that their evidence supported Hering's law and differed from other electromyographic investigators both in the interpretation of Hering's law and supporting electromyographic data.

From the figures of their paper, it appears that the cocontraction of the horizontal recti during asymmetric convergence was elicited in the vicinity of the near point, where divergence occurred. The studies of intermittent exotropia in Figures 4 to 10 were obtained by fixating a near target; in short, all their studies appear to have been obtained at the near point where the mechanism of central adjustment of opposing vergence and version innervation is critically strained. There is no doubt that cocontraction may occur at or near the breakpoint. This increased activity may not persist following the restoration of fusion as is seen in Figure 6 where the right medial rectus, following a phase of cocontraction, appears to revert to the level of innervation existing before fusion was obtained. The cocontraction, therefore, may be a transient phenomenon. Furthermore, the decrease in activity in the stationary eye with break in fusion was, according to the authors, not found as consistently or seen as readily as the increased activity with refusion. Thus, in Figure 8, there is no change of activity in the right medial rectus when fusion is broken. They stated that this eye always showed an observable increase in this muscle during refusion and they were unable to explain the discrepancy. In Figure 10, where a quick movement is made by the stationary eye at the start of rapid asymmetric convergence, the return of the innervation to the level existing before fusion was obtained is quite evident in the right medial rectus.

In the discussion of this paper, Blodi[22] reaffirmed the principle of central adjustment of opposing innervations and cited additional experiments of asymmetric convergence in different directions of gaze, always with identical results.

Tamler,[134] in the discussion, made the statement that if one performs asymmetric convergence with the moving eye occluded so that the only stimulus the stationary eye gets is accommodative, then there is no change in the horizontal rectus muscles of the stationary eye. This, in itself, is a refutation of their basic position, since accommodative vergence so elicited must still require an opposing version innervation to neutralize it in the non-moving eye. This, according to their thesis, should be visible as cocontraction; yet they report that it does not occur.

In the discussion, Alpern[5] stated that he was quite sure that the changes described by the authors would be encountered on sudden asymmetric convergence shifts, but doubted that they would be seen in the gradual type of asymmetric convergence. He also had reported the absence of movement of the fixing eye in monocular asymmetric convergence by electro-oculography. This subject will be discussed further subsequently.

In 1959, D'Esposito, Serra, and Ambrosio[56] reviewed some of the ocular electromyographic literature in Italian.

In 1959, Tamler, Marg, and Jampolsky[130] described coactivity of human extraocular muscles in following movements. Electromyography with electrode insertion in the four rectus muscles of an eye recorded no increased electric activity of auxiliary muscles during slow vertical and horizontal following movements in planes through the primary position. The absence of electric alteration in auxiliary muscles during rotations did not preclude their contributing to the action since the function of a muscle varies with the position of the eye. In these findings the authors confirmed the previous conclusions of Breinin.[31]

Marg, Jampolsky, and Tamler[100] reported on the elements of human extraocular electromyography. This paper is an elementary description of the equipment and technique of electromyography with a brief discussion of the neurophysiologic principles involved. The use of a 2-M./sec. camera speed is a worth-while addition since extraocular motor units may sometimes require such high speeds for adequate display of the wave form.

Buchthal's suggestion[43] of the term "subunit" for the fibers that are recorded in unit activity was mentioned with the comment that this may not be the case in extraocular muscle because of the low innervation ratio. The authors also stressed that for the identification of single units not only are the frequency and height necessary, but also the wave form. They stated that eye movements of less than 8° cannot be demonstrated in the electromyogram. The advantages of multiple channel recording are as follows: blinks can be revealed since they register on all channels; distinctive activity of a single muscle stands out more clearly from artifacts; instances of coactivity or cocontraction can readily be measured by multiple channels whereas a single or even a dual channel apparatus does not give a complete picture; binocular function can be more directly and readily measured. They further stated that human extraocular electromyography is an important research tool, but that its clinical value is limited chiefly to neuro-ophthalmologic diagnosis and prognosis. The selection of patients must be made with care. Generally, children cannot be examined and the personality of adults must be such that they are willing to undergo what to most persons is a somewhat frightening and not entirely painless procedure. Elderly patients occasionally get subconjunctival hemorrhages. They further stated that limitation of eye movement by paralysis or mechanical restriction can usually be diagnosed clinically and that electromyography merely confirms these findings. Therefore, electromyograms are neither necessary nor helpful in usual practical motility problems. Overactivity cannot be distinguished from underactivity, since the amplitude of the trace is largely dependent upon the insertion. A moderate or severe paresis or paralysis is obvious without the aid of electrical techniques. These statements deserve further study and will be discussed below.

Jampolsky, Tamler, and Marg[77] reported upon artifacts and normal variations in human ocular electromyography. In connection with normal variations, they pointed out the following.

1. The degree of activity will vary, depending upon electrode muscle relationships; hence, sampling differences may alter the amplitude of the electromyogram. The strength of a muscle contraction, therefore, cannot be inferred from electromyographic data except in marked neurogenic disease. They do not believe that spastic esotropia can be diagnosed from the amplitude of the electromyogram.

2. Recording activity from more than one muscle with a single electrode may result in confusion, and they stated that in practice this is restricted to the electrode insertion near the crossing of the inferior oblique and inferior rectus muscles. Recording from both muscles could simulate the picture of anomalous innervation.

3. Electrode movement may result in the recording of activity in one direction of gaze which alters when, because of the movement, the tip of the needle works out of the muscle. Such displacements could be picked up by reinsertion of the electrode with recovery of electric activity. They pointed out that this occurs very infrequently. Electrode movement *per se* does not alter the recording.

4. The measured time relationships of electric activity between muscles vary. Different electrode positions will exhibit a different time of onset, although the pattern of activity in the various muscle positions will be similar.

In connection with artifacts they pointed out the following.

1. Television artifacts have a characteristic wave form and duration (1.25 msec. and a frequency of 60 pulses per sec.). With inadequate screening, television artifacts may be recorded in the electromyogram. Of considerable interest was their demonstration that such artifacts may wax and wane with the effort and amplitude exhibited in the electromyogram, thus simulating motor unit activity. They emphasized that fast film sweeps are necessary for proper analysis and interpretation, and suggested that such artifacts may be similar to evidence given in support of anomalous innervation.

2. Artifacts of base-line movement. Shifts of the base line sometimes resembling motor unit activity may occur. At the beginning or end of a fast eye movement such artifactual shifts may be misinterpreted as summated electric activity. They suggested that fast film sweeps are

required to display the character of the innervation. Eyelid movement may cause such artifacts, as is seen during blinks.

3. Orbicularis muscle activity may also be recorded as an increase in activity of the extraocular muscles.

4. Artifacts recorded with poor electrode insertion or low-amplitude recording. Such records are considered especially prone to demonstration of artifacts.

5. Improper shielding and inadequate amplifier balance may allow the recording of extraneous electric activity, intrinsic in the individual or extrinsic in the environment. They stated that some of these rhythmic changes may be confused with spindle pattern activity.

6. They stated that other waves of activity may occur in muscle paresis or exophthalmos. (These are obviously not artifactual in nature.)

7. Overloading of the amplifier or oscillation of the amplifier may produce recording difficulties. (These are usually quite obvious.)

8. Variations in film speed at the beginning and end may produce an apparent change in frequency of units which is, in fact, a reflection of the inertia of the camera employed.

In their summary, Jampolsky *et al.* pointed out that eye movement or position may not be extracted from an electromyogram, with any degree of certainty; that is, one may have electromyographic changes without eye movement and one may have eye movement without electromyographic changes. They criticized the electromyographic concepts expressed in the literature of spastic esotropia, retractory nystagmus, anomalous innervation, Hering's law, and the divergence mechanism as described by Breinin and others.

It is an elementary fact known to all workers in electrophysiology that one can produce virtually any desired electric pattern by manipulation of the equipment or recording conditions. The fact that the authors have recorded spontaneous or induced artifactual phenomena resembling patterns described by others does not establish an identity between the two.

In a report in 1959, Tamler, Jampolsky, and Marg[133] briefly reviewed some of the contributions made by this technique in strabismus with a criticism of the results of others.

McLean and Norton,[103] in 1959, reported on unilateral lid retraction without exophthalmos. They pointed out that unilateral lid retraction is associated with thyroid dysfunction and that this cannot be innervational in origin. One of the points in evidence was the levator electromyogram of such patients showing complete inhibition of activity in gaze down with the retention of lid retraction. The electromyography in these cases was performed by Breinin. They concluded that the retraction was secondary to changes in the levator muscle.

In 1959, Sears, Teasdall, and Stone[122] reported an electromyographic study of stretch effects in human extraocular muscle. Eight patients were investigated prior to enucleation of one eye. The action potentials were recorded in primary and lateral gaze from one horizontal rectus muscle and the effect of passive stretch observed. With the eyes in the primary position the action potentials were unchanged by disinsertion or manual pull. During agonist contraction, however, stretch of the agonist itself, the antagonist, or yoke muscle, produced a decrease in the frequency and amplitude of its discharges. This inhibitory effect was not observed when stretch was applied to the muscles of the eye which had a previous retrobulbar alcohol injection or to the involved muscle in a patient with a third nerve palsy. They suggested that the extraocular muscles of man have receptors which can be stimulated by passive stretch. Such inhibitory reflexes have not been encountered by any other investigators.

In 1959, Kornblueth, Jampolsky, Tamler, and Marg[83] reported an electromyographic study of the activity of the oculorotary muscles during tonometry and tonography. Nineteen patients were studied. Holding a tonometer near or on the eye consistently caused a cocontraction of the extraocular muscles which was simultaneous in both eyes. This reaction was not necessarily accompanied by contraction of the orbicularis and occurred also after akinesia of the lids. This is considered a protective or fright reaction of central origin and is dependent on sight as it did not occur in blind or nearly blind subjects or in patients under general anesthesia.

Tonography showed an initial cocontraction of the extraocular muscles which diminished over the course of four minutes. The authors suggested that the changes in tonus of the muscles caused by tonometry or tonography may alter the intraocular pressure in both eyes, introducing some inaccuracies in these procedures. The massage effect of the muscle contraction, therefore, could be a factor in producing a steep initial fall of the tonographic curve and the ophthalmotonic consensual reflex. Strong, manual pressure upon the globe through the closed lids evoked a cocontraction of the muscles limited to the side of the pressed globe. They attributed this to a local peripheral adjustment of the muscles to take up the slack produced by the enophthalmos. Nasal or temporal displacement of the globe did not produce this reaction. (No such adjustment of innervation has been encountered in man or animals by any investigators and one would expect either no change or a decreased activity with enophthalmos.) The bilateral cocontraction was considered a manifestation of Hering's law of equal distribution of nerve impulses.

Tamler, Marg, Jampolsky, and Nawratzki,[131] in 1959, reported on the electromyography of human saccadic eye movement. During a saccade there was a heightened burst of activity of the agonist, inhibition of the antagonist, and cocontraction of the auxiliary extraocular muscles. The duration of saccades of different degrees of excursion was measured by simultaneous electromyography and electro-oculography. They presented evidence to show that saccadic eye movements are not ballistic. The evidence for the cocontraction of auxiliary muscles is conflicting since it was present at some times and not others. In particular, it was not present in a poor electrode insertion, the very situation in which, they repeatedly state, artifacts are common. Increased activity of an inferior oblique during rapid horizontal movements of the eye had also been noted by Bjork.[19] The authors affirmed the non-ballistic nature of eye movement previously demonstrated by Breinin[36] in 1958. The authors took issue with Miller[106] concerning the nature of the saccade and denied that there is an initial burst of activity followed by a more uniform, orderly pattern. They stated that there is no apparent variation in unit activity during the saccade. They further disputed the occurrence of afterbursts with fixational correction.

In 1959, Miller[107] reported upon the electromyography of the vergence movement. Six normal individuals were studied. Of particular interest was his observation that after the insertion of multiple electrodes erratic eye movements were produced. The author concluded the following.

1. Convergence utilizes more motor units than saccadic movement of the same magnitude.

2. Part of the motor units is different in the two patterns.

3. Divergence activity resembles saccadic movement and the pattern is different from convergent motion.

4. *Sudden* asymmetric convergence is accompanied by a saccadic burst in agonists, followed by a convergent pattern in both medial recti.

5. No increase in cocontraction of horizontal antagonists is noted with *slow* asymmetric convergence on an approaching target, until the near point of convergence is approached.

Convergence differed from saccadic movement, having a more

gradual increment at the onset followed by changing activity for almost
a second. There did not seem to be any corrective adjustments and
the activity gradually declined. Several of the figures showed a spindle
pattern of innervation for convergence. Single motor units showed a
similar pattern. Divergence was found to consist of two types. The
first showed cocontraction of the medial and lateral rectus; a spindle
pattern appeared in the lateral rectus coincident with a saccadic
burst in the medial rectus as the eye diverged. The second form of
divergence was marked by inhibition of the medial rectus coincident
with a saccade in the lateral rectus, with a regular reciprocating
pattern following until a stable state was reached. Secondary bursts
of saccadic type were also seen in divergence. Sudden asymmetric
convergence was characterized by a saccadic burst in yoke muscles
followed by a convergence pattern in the medial recti. The supposedly
stationary eye showed similar changes, with a saccade in the lateral
rectus followed by a convergence pattern in the medial rectus. On the
other hand, if the asymmetric convergence was gradual, by following
a slowly approaching target, no alteration in the electromyograms was
noted until the object approached the near point of convergence when
cocontraction began. This occurred in one instance at 6 cm. from the
eye, or about 16 meter angles. Divergence then occurred in one of the
two forms described.

The author observed that there is no doubt that divergence is active.
He considered that the two forms of divergence may be on a sampling
basis, since only a small area of ocular muscle was surveyed at a given
instance.

Using the single motor unit technique, movements as small as $2\frac{1}{2}°$
could be discerned. The author considered cocontraction as a normal
variant of divergence and suggested that this represented the beginning
of divergence under the conditions of a slowly advancing stimulus. He
further observed that he had found cocontraction in normal subjects
at the near point of symmetric convergence and that in subjects with
a remote near point of convergence, this simultaneous increase
occurred at a greater distance for both symmetric and asymmetric
convergence.

Tamler, Jampolsky, and Marg[132] reported an electromyographic
study of following movements of the eye between tertiary positions.
The eyes were tested in vertical and horizontal planes at the limit of
the excursions. They concluded that in horizontal following movements
between tertiary positions the vertical recti are consistently more active
in abduction than in adduction, whereas the reverse is true for the

inferior oblique. The horizontal recti manifested no consistent pattern of electric alteration from subject to subject in vertical tertiary plane following movements, showing in some cases alterations of activity and in others none. The greater activity of the vertical recti in abduction and of the obliques in adduction in tertiary positions confirmed the previous findings of Breinin.[26,31]

They attributed the failure of Momosse[109] to find changes of these muscles to the fact that he recorded activity only at the 23° position. The changes reported did not occur during vertical and horizontal movements through the primary position. They were unable to explain the variations in horizontal recti activity in vertical movements into tertiary positions, but suggested a mechanism of peripheral proprioceptive feedback as a possibility. They criticized the suggestion of Breinin[34] that the A and V syndromes can be explained, in part, on the basis of changes in activity of the horizontal recti during vertical movements. They suggested that the mere presence of increased activity of the muscles may only reflect the new position of the eye rather than telling how or why the eye moved to this new position. Because of the normal variation in activity of horizontal recti in tertiary plane movements, they considered it misleading to draw conclusions regarding causation of the A or V syndromes without at least adequate sampling. These points will be discussed below.

A case report on progressive dystrophic external ophthalmoplegia with abiotrophic fundus changes was presented by Thorson and Bell[136] in 1959. An electromyogram of the lateral rectus muscles showed that, despite almost complete immobility of the eyes and ptosis, there was abundant recruitment of low-voltage motor units on effort. A normal reciprocity pattern was found and no evidences of denervation were present. Electroretinograms were markedly abnormal and a muscle biopsy of the right lateral rectus showed characteristic dystrophic changes. They considered such cases as examples of multiple abiotrophies.

INSTRUMENTATION AND TECHNIQUE (FIGURE 1)

Critical electrophysiologic work requires high standards of instrumentation. The very low electromyographic potentials may be suitably amplified by pre-amplifiers having a frequency response of from a fraction of a cycle up to 10,000 cycles or higher. The amplified bioelectric signal is then displayed upon the face of a cathode-ray oscilloscope containing one or preferably two beams. Versatility may

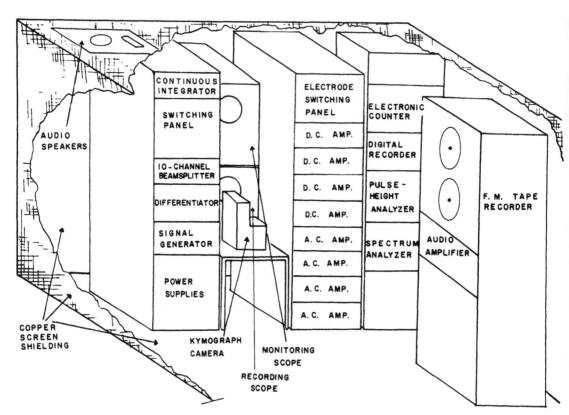

FIGURE 1. EQUIPMENT LAYOUT FOR ELECTROMYOGRAPHY

be increased by the use of electronic switches to provide multichannel records. The electric traces are photographed by a moving-film, 35-mm. variable-speed Grass camera. Film speeds of 10 cm. per sec. up to 1 or even 2 M. per sec. are used. Time marks of 100 cycles per sec. and 1,000 cycles per sec. should be available as well as amplitude calibration markers. The latter may be either a square wave or sine wave. The patient must be tested in an electrically shielded room to prevent the recording of extraneous electric potentials. Suitable electrically shielded rooms are commercially available. Auxiliary apparatus helpful but not essential in electromyographic studies are integrators, differentiators, pulse counters, frequency analyzers, and, in particular, a sensitive magnetic tape system which can, with fidelity, record the electric activity of the extraocular muscles. The tapes then permit future study, as desired, of the live electric signals. An audio-amplifier is an essential in electromyographic recording since the signals are more readily heard than seen. In some cases the diagnosis can be made from the sound of the electric activity. The pre-amplifiers should be capacity coupled, although DC amplifiers working on short time constants are also usable. Two or more channels of pre-amplifiers should be available.

Electrodes may be either monopolar or concentric. The former is readily fabricated, cheap, and convenient, but requires an extra, indifferent electrode placement. The concentric electrode of Adrian and Bronk provides a more limited field of pickup and can be used with advantage in the exploration of small muscle areas. No indifferent electrode is required. The more selective concentric electrode can be refined to almost microelectrode sensitivity.

For general ocular use, 30- or 31-gauge, 1-inch-long needles are employed. A fine (40-gauge or higher) insulated wire is inserted down the bore of the needle and only the tip left uninsulated. The pickup area of the electrode then lies between the uncoated barrel end and the exposed tip of the inner wire. Many structural variations are possible to alter the electrode characteristics.

The patient must always be electrically grounded and this can be conveniently done with a surface disk electrode such as is used in electroencephalography. A simple copper earring affixed to the lobe of the patient's ear is very satisfactory. The impedance of the ground electrode can be decreased by the use of electrode paste. The shielded cage, the equipment in it, and the patient must all be connected to the same ground, otherwise ground loops will be formed giving rise to 60-cycle AC interference. The patient is placed on a table or preferably in a reclining chair such as the Barcalounger. A few drops of topical pontocaine, 0.5 percent, are all that is required for ocular anesthesia. For insertion of electrodes into the recti muscles, the conjunctiva is picked up over the tendon of the muscle with fine forceps. The electrode is inserted and in one or two motions plunged into the belly of the muscle in a direction almost parallel to the muscle axis. The audio-monitor and the oscilloscope will exhibit the signal when the electrode is in proper position. With experience, the placement becomes quite simple. A blepharostat may be used but is not necessary. It does help to limit lid artifacts but can be dispensed with if care is employed in the study of the patient. Exposure keratitis can be severe in patients whose lids are held open for long periods. Topical methyl cellulose may help to cut down corneal drying.

The inferior oblique muscle is easily available through the skin at the medial aspect of the inferior orbital margin. The electrode is plunged through the skin into the muscle near its origin. With experience it can be placed in the muscle belly with one or two thrusts. No anesthesia of any kind is necessary in this procedure.

The superior oblique muscle is difficult to locate but a long needle electrode can be inserted through the upper lid or through the superior conjunctival fornix and into the muscle.

The levator is best reached through the superior conjunctival fornix after double eversion of the lid on a Desmarre's hook.

The electrodes may be sterilized in zephiran. This does not obviate the possibility of transmitting hepatotoxic viruses. Electrodes can be made which can be autoclaved and these, no doubt, are safer.

Following electromyography an antibiotic ointment is placed in the eye. Usually no patch is required.

The question of how many electrodes to insert in extraocular muscles is important. One electrode may suffice to give all the information required for a diagnosis. In kinesiologic studies, however, it is better to have two electrodes which can be placed in antagonistic muscles. With two electrodes one can determine the essential innervational characteristics of the extraocular muscles, although not always in one maneuver. By performing serial studies in different muscle sets the total picture can be put together beyond question.

Marg, Jampolsky, and Tamler[100] have advocated the use of multi-channel recording with electrode insertions in four, six, or perhaps eight extraocular muscles in one or both eyes. They routinely employ at least four insertions, sometimes in four muscles of one eye, sometimes distributed between the two eyes. What are the virtues of this technique? It is true that it presents a simultaneous picture of activity in many muscles which from a theoretical viewpoint is desirable; however, it is very questionable whether the muscles following such multiple electrode placements are in a normal physiological state. There is evidence that after even two placements fixation may become erratic, and certainly after multiple placements this has been noted. Vision tends to become blurry following such electrode placements with disturbances of accommodation. Technically, control of multiple placements is very difficult, particularly during movements of the eyes. The technique constitutes a *tour de force* in the hands of the above authors which one can only admire. Instrumentationally, it requires a multichannel system which, of course, is expensive and not generally available.

The insertion of an electrode, although relatively atraumatic, can on occasion be painful. The insertion of multiple electrodes tends to be even more painful with a much heightened incidence of subconjunctival hemorrhages, exposure keratitis, and other undesired effects. One instance of subcapsular hemorrhage has been encountered at surgery following electromyography. From the purely scientific viewpoint one can obtain all the findings necessary with two electrodes. Since the technical complications, trauma, and discomfort to the subject are tremendously increased by such multiple electrode placements, and since fixation and vision may be compromised, the multiple electrode technique must be considered unnecessary and probably inadvisable.

For quantification of the electromyogram either a discontinuous or a continuous integrator may be employed; each has its advantages and failings. Integration consists of the summing up of the electric activity of the signal and its display in a simple fashion. The discontinuous integrator may include a differentiating circuit which converts motor units into pulses. These are fed into an electronic counter which totals them and may even print out this frequency information automatically. An excellent tape system is the Ampex FM multichannel unit which has a frequency response from DC to 10,000 cycles and tape speeds of 1⅞ to 60 in. per sec. With this equipment it is possible to tape signals at high speed and play them back at any desired rate. A reduction factor of 30:1 is available. If desired, the electromyogram can be played back through this reduction system into an ink writer. In general, ink writers are not suitable for electromyography because the inertia of the pens does not permit them to follow the very fast potentials of extraocular muscle. This difficulty is obviated by the tape reduction system.

A microphone connected to a separate channel is necessary in connection with the tape record to monitor the electric signal. A coding mark is helpful to indicate specific events in the electric record. For coding film in the Grass camera, a simple, inexpensive system[145] has been devised employing a Nixie neon bulb with numbers from one to ten which are photographed before each record.

GENERAL PRINCIPLES OF ELECTROMYOGRAPHY

NORMAL ELECTRIC ACTIVITY (SEE FIGURE 2, A AND B)

The electromyogram is a record of the electric discharge of muscle, not of nerve. The physical substrate for this discharge is the anatomical motor unit consisting of the neuron cell body, its axon, and the group of muscle fibers innervated by that axon. When the electric impulse sweeps down the axon and strikes the motor endplates, all the muscle fibers discharge synchronously. The integrated voltage of this discharge constitutes the electric motor unit.[43,54]

The amplitude of a motor unit is dependent upon many factors, chief of which is the relation of the recording electrode to the discharging fibers. The further removed the electrode is from the unit, the lower the amplitude; the closer it is, the higher the amplitude. Also, the more spatially distributed are the muscle fibers of the unit, the smaller will be the electric energy captured in the receptive field of the recording electrode. The shape or wave form of the motor unit will vary with the geometry of the electrode-unit relationship. When the electrode is not in immediate contact with the discharging unit, it may reflect only the envelope of electric activity; whereas, in the immediate vicinity of the unit (subunit), it will exhibit a spike. The motor unit spike with good electrode position is a diphasic wave, that is, with an initial positivity (downward deflection) followed by a negativity (upward deflection) characteristic of traveling waves. Occasionally, the wave form is triphasic (source-sink-source), showing the modification of the body as a volume conductor. A monophasic wave may result from asymmetric positioning of the electrode. Multiphasic or polyphasic potentials are occasionally found in normal skeletal muscle (3 percent) but rarely occur in normal extraocular muscle. Motor units of peripheral skeletal muscle have an amplitude of 100 μv. to 2 or 3 mv. and a duration of 5–10 msec. They exhibit a frequency of firing of some 5–30 per sec. By contrast, extraocular motor units have a much lower amplitude, averaging 20 to 200 μv. but occasionally reaching as high as 400 to 600 μv. Their duration is much shorter, averaging 1–2 msec. Their rate of firing is very much higher, reaching several hundred

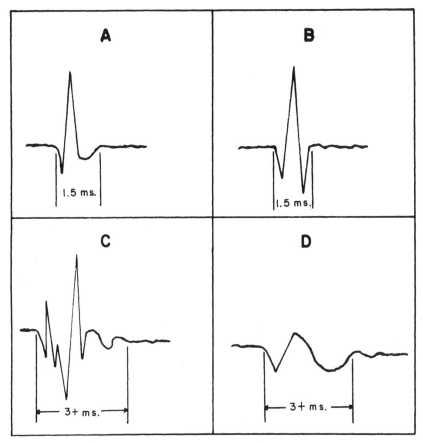

FIGURE 2. NORMAL AND ABNORMAL ELECTRIC ACTIVITY

A, diphasic action potential; B, triphasic (source-sink-source) action potential; C, polyphasic configuration; D, myasthenic muscle action potential.

discharges per second and they can recruit faster than peripheral motor units.

The basis of these differences lies in the composition of the anatomical motor unit. The peripheral skeletal muscle unit consists of one axon distributed to 100–200 muscle fibers.[24,46,135] The extraocular muscle motor unit, on the other hand, has a very much lower innervation ratio with one axon distributed to only 5–10 muscle fibers.[135] If the muscle fibers are considered the batteries of the unit, which are added up in series to form the total integrated voltage, it is obvious that the extraocular units must have a very much lower potential. Low innervation ratios are characteristic of muscles involved in delicate, precise, finely graded functions such as characterize the movements of the eye. Large innervation ratios are found in muscles with gross function such as the large limb muscles.

Insertion potentials, brief bursts of high frequency, may be elicited on insertion of the electrode. Irritation of the muscle by electrode movement may also evoke discharges.

Despite the existence of tonus, skeletal muscle at rest evinces no recordable electric potentials. This, however, is not true of the extraocular muscles which rarely are electrically silent.[14,26,84] Nerve and muscle augment their activity in several ways. The frequency of discharge of units increases and additional units are recruited, some of which are of larger amplitude with higher thresholds.

In peripheral skeletal muscle, the electric pattern goes from resting silence to moderate firing on minimal effort to profuse firing on maximum effort. In extraocular muscles, the initial pattern of response to effort is the discharge of small single units which increase in frequency and number to form a more complex (mixed) pattern, eventually resulting in the so-called interference pattern in which the overlapping of activity prevents identification of individual units. The overlapping discharges integrate in amplitude but exhibit numerous humps or buttons, indicating that several potentials are involved. Fast oscilloscope sweeps or camera speeds are necessary to separate units and to identify the wave form properly. Although only a small area of muscle is sampled by the electrode, the activity seems fairly representative of the entire muscle; however, the time course of such activity may vary with electrode position.[34,77] The differences reflect the asynchronous discharge of motor units which permits gradation of muscle activity and smoothness of contraction. There is no evidence of rotation of units in extraocular muscle.

Some electrode movement must occur in ocular rotations. There is, however, surprising constancy of electrode unit relationship since frequently one can pick up the identical unit at the same place despite large rotations of the globe. It is, nevertheless, possible to displace the electrode from a particular muscle recording area with consequent alterations of the signal. In general, slight electrode movement does not appear to affect the record.

ABNORMAL ELECTRIC ACTIVITY (SEE FIGURES 2, C AND D, AND 3)

Polyphasic units consist of a series of oscillations which represent the non-synchronized discharge of a motor unit. As has been mentioned, they occur occasionally in normal peripheral skeletal muscle

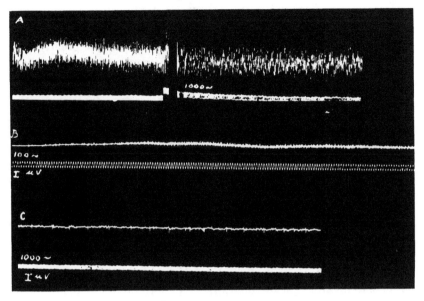

FIGURE 3. OCULAR ELECTROMYOGRAM

A, normal medial rectus; B, myopathy; C, lower motor neuron disease.

(3 percent) but are quite rare in normal extraocular muscle.[15,19] They are thought to result from temporal or spatial dispersion of the nerve impulse and may indicate a lesion which disrupts the synchronous discharge of the muscle fibers of the unit. They frequently occur following denervation or during reinnervation of a muscle.

Some of the most diagnostic findings of electromyography are the fibrillation potentials of denervation.[55,62,141] These are considered to be the output of a single muscle fiber having an amplitude in peripheral muscle of 50–100 μv., a duration of 1–2 msec., and a frequency of 2–10 per sec. They occur independently of volition, appearing about 2 to 3 weeks after denervation. They occur while the muscle is at rest. If recovery ensues, their number decreases while there is a gradual development of polyphasic potentials which, in turn, give place to normal motor units. A certain number of fibrillations and polyphasics may persist up to and after complete clinical recovery. A slow positive wave potential of 4–8-msec. duration may also be seen in denervation. It is obvious that denervation potentials resemble closely normal extraocular motor units and it should be noted that they are infrequently recognized in extraocular muscle lesions.[17,26,78,108]

It should also be noted that 20–30 percent of peripheral muscle denervation is unaccompanied by fibrillation.[43] Fibrillation may persist for many years ending only with fibrosis and atrophy of the muscle.

The frequency of firing of units in pareses may increase greatly over the normal rates in an apparent attempt to compensate for the weakness. A tendency to grouping of units may occur in neurogenic lesions.[78]

Reinnervation potentials of long duration may reach very high amplitudes. They are particularly common in the misdirection syndrome.[29]

Conduction block paralysis results from compression of a nerve without denervation. There is electric silence at rest and on volition, without fibrillation. Tourniquet paralysis is an example of such a block.

In the peripheral musculature, upper motor neuron lesions may reveal simultaneous activity of antagonists, synchrony of firing, and disturbances of reciprocity.

In neuropathic lesions, there is a decrease in total unit activity with consequent loss of the interference pattern on effort. Recruitment is irregular and poorly sustained while the remaining units may vary greatly in amplitude.[62]

Myopathic lesions such as muscular dystrophy or myositis exhibit abundant unit discharges of low amplitude on effort, units of shortened duration and the presence of many polyphasics.[43] These characteristics are considered to result from the destruction of muscle fibers, the batteries of the unit, with loss of integrated voltage. The intact axons are fired more frequently to compensate for the muscle weakness. Interference patterns are thus readily produced in myopathic muscle. These features are not always encountered in extraocular myopathies.[112]

In the determination of lesions of muscles, it is important to make several electrode placements to sample different areas. Inadequate sampling may result in erroneous interpretations.

HUMAN EXTRAOCULAR ELECTROMYOGRAPHY

KINESIOLOGY

INNERVATIONAL CHARACTERISTICS (SEE FIGURES 4 TO 7). The response of the extraocular muscles to nerve stimulation in animals has demonstrated their great rapidity of contraction,[51] the short twitch duration being associated with a very high frequency required for tetanic fusion. High rates of motor unit firing would be expected and are found in the extraocular muscles of man.[14] A striking finding in extraocular muscle

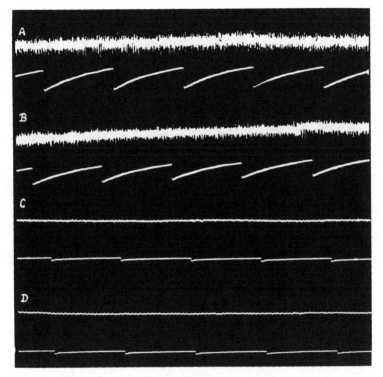

FIGURE 4. ELECTROMYOGRAM OF LEFT INFERIOR OBLIQUE
Fields of gaze: A, up and in; B, up and out; C, down and in; D, down
and out.

is the presence of constant tonic activity in the primary position during the waking state.[14,26] This is in marked contrast to peripheral skeletal muscle, which is electrically silent at rest. The activity diminishes as the eye rotates out of the field of action of the muscle and may be reduced to the firing of a few units or none at all in the most extreme position of gaze. On rotation into the field of action, individual motor units of low amplitude appear, which increase their frequency of discharge as the rotation continues. In addition, new units appear, some of which are of higher amplitude. Some units appear to have a specific range of activity,[86-88] appearing and disappearing within a certain number of degrees of rotation. Upon reaching the primary position, the activity may become so dense as to be an interference pattern, although one may frequently distinguish individual units superimposed upon a denser firing background (mixed pattern). Upon moving further into the field of action, the interference pattern becomes

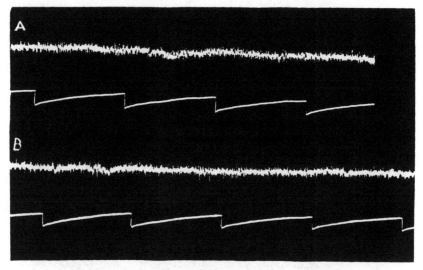

FIGURE 5. LEFT INFERIOR OBLIQUE, NO CHANGE IN HORIZONTAL PLANE
EMG, *above*; integration, *below*. A, adduction; B, abduction.

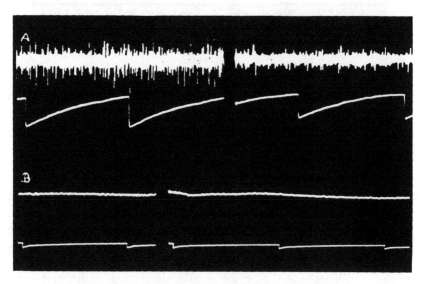

FIGURE 6. ELECTROMYOGRAM OF RIGHT SUPERIOR RECTUS
Fields of gaze: A, up and out (*left*), up and in (*right*); B, down and in (*left*), down and out (*right*).

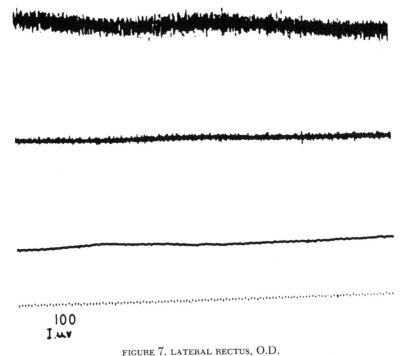

100
I µv

FIGURE 7. LATERAL RECTUS, O.D.

Upper tracing records field of maximum activity (abduction); *middle tracing*, primary position with rhythmic motor unit activity; *lower tracing*, inhibition in the adducted position. Time in 100 cycles.

more marked with a large increase of higher-amplitude potentials. Many potentials summate, producing notches, humps, or buttons which can only be separated by fast oscilloscope sweeps or film speed. Upon reaching the extreme limit of rotation on further effort, the electric activity may actually fall off with the appearance of broader potentials. This, in some instances, may be due to displacement of the electrode from the active muscle area. In other instances, it may represent an innervational change possibly due to inhibition. This fall-off may be seen in the integrated electromyogram[37,110] and in the differentiated frequency count.[37]

The auditory accompaniment of version movements varies from the popping activity produced by single units out of the field of gaze to the roaring activity of the interference pattern.

The smallest amount of movement distinguishable in the ocular electromyogram is about five degrees. Somewhat smaller rotations are discernible with fine electrodes.[106]

The discharge frequency of a single unit is quite constant during fixation of the gaze but varies as the gaze varies.[87] With rates of firing below 30 per sec., considerable variation may be encountered in the firing rate of a single unit. The behavior of single units in antagonistic muscles, although generally reciprocal, may exhibit deviations from this principle. Occasionally, units in the antagonist may increase their rate of discharge despite movement out of their field; the possibility of this being due to a stretch reflex has been suggested.[88]

Some Japanese authors,[89,90] employing a technique whose validity is not clearly established, described slow and fast rhythms in the firing patterns of extraocular muscle. These rhythms are demonstrated in individual motor units by means of Fourier analysis and are considered to be the same as Piper rhythm in peripheral skeletal muscle. The frequency spectra demonstrate a mode value of frequency of slow rhythm in the primary position between 70 and 100 cycles per sec., with fast rhythm in the adducted position between 150 and 250 cycles per sec. These values correlate well with the firing rate of motor units in corresponding positions.[128] The slow and fast rhythm are considered to represent the activity of tonic and kinetic units.[84,121] Slow rhythm has been described from the 30° abducted to the extremely adducted position of the eye. Fast rhythm appeared only at the adducted positions over 30°, when it was superimposed on the slow rhythm.

Other studies of discharge rhythms have been made by Japanese investigators which demonstrate fluctuations that do not correlate well with any natural phenomena.[79] The effect of flicker light stimulation of the retina upon the extraocular muscles has been investigated. It is said to elicit muscle potentials suggesting the arousal reaction and produce high-frequency motor unit discharge in the absence of appreciable eye movement.[80]

LEVATOR AND ORBICULARIS. The behavior of the levator palpebrae superioris is similar to that of the recti muscles. Although it has been stated that the motor unit of the levator is somewhat longer in duration,[15] there does not appear to be any marked difference between its units and those of other extraocular muscles. The innervational pattern is quite similar, ranging from an absence of innervation on gaze down, although occasionally low-amplitude single units may still fire, to an interference pattern on gaze up.

The behavior of the levator in the baboon[68] and in man is identical and it has been shown to participate in vertical nystagmus innervation along with the vertical extraocular muscles.

The action potentials of the orbicularis oculi[29] are intermediate in character between extraocular muscle and peripheral skeletal musculature. Polyphasic potentials are more frequently encountered just as in peripheral muscle, and the orbicularis at rest is electrically silent. Reciprocity is clearly demonstrable between the orbicularis and the levator in forced closure of the eye.[18,26,68] When the lids are lowered, the levator activity progressively decreases, reaching electric silence or thereabouts in gaze down. During this time the orbicularis does not fire. However, when the eyes are forcibly closed, the orbicularis fires briskly and the levator is inhibited. During blinks the orbicularis fires in bursts with accompanying inhibition in the levator which precedes and follows the burst of the orbicularis by a short interval.[68] Activity of the orbicularis should not be confused with the firing of the extraocular muscles when placing the electrode through the skin into the inferior oblique. Orbicularis activity due to lid squeezing is a potential source of interference, but such activity would be seen in all leads of the electromyogram.

RECIPROCAL INNERVATION (SEE FIGURE 8). It has been clearly shown in animals[23,81,82,94,124,125] and in man[16,26] that antagonistic extraocular

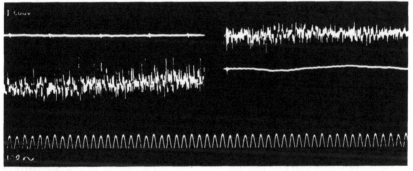

FIGURE 8. RECIPROCAL RELATIONSHIP, LATERAL RECTI OF THE TWO EYES
Upper tracing, O.S.; *lower tracing*, O.D. On extreme gaze right there is marked activity of the lateral rectus O.D. with almost complete inhibition of the left lateral rectus. On extreme gaze left, the left lateral rectus fires maximally, while there is complete inhibition of the right lateral rectus.

muscles usually observe Sherrington's principle of reciprocal innervation. Augmentation of activity in the agonist is accompanied by a concomitant, parallel decrement of activity in the antagonist.

The law of reciprocity is beautifully exemplified in both direct and contralateral antagonists. Synergists show a parallel increase of activity. Yoke muscles demonstrate the same pattern of augmentation in gaze into their field and inhibition in gaze away from their field. Reciprocal innervation is clearly demonstrated in jerky nystagmus. Here, the burst of activity in the agonist is accompanied by an abrupt inhibition of the antagonist. In pendular nystagmus, the activity reciprocally waxes and wanes smoothly in agonist and antagonist.

The exception to the reciprocity law, cocontraction (the simultaneous increase in activity of antagonists), may occur at the near point of convergence,[129] in association with divergence,[26,107] during the fright reaction to an object closely approximated to the eye[37,83] and during neurological disturbances.[29,36,94] Individual units may deviate from the reciprocity pattern but this is infrequent.[86,88] Cocontraction possibly occurs in antagonistic muscles during a rapid saccadic movement in a plane at right angles to their line of action.[130] Such cocontraction disappears at the termination of the rapid movement. Cocontraction may occur simultaneously in both eyes when a tonometer is suspended above or on one eye. This reaction depends upon vision. It may constitute a source of error during tonography, but the practical significance of the observation has not been established.[83]

The term "coactivity" has been used in place of cocontraction,[130] but it is a substitute which adds nothing to the description of the physiological event and which is no more meaningful than the well-known term, cocontraction. Although cocontraction does occur in the extraocular muscles, its role is very much subordinate to that of reciprocal innervation which obtains throughout the widest range of physiologic movement.

AUXILIARY ROTATORS (SEE FIGURES 4–6). The auxiliary role of the vertical muscles in horizontal gaze and of the horizontal muscles in vertical gaze has been investigated.[31,109,132] The electric activity of vertical muscles during horizontal gaze through the primary position demonstrates no significant change. Similarly, the electric activity of horizontal muscles in vertical gaze through the primary position shows no significant change. Therefore, the vertical movers are not active accessory abductors or adductors, nor are the horizontal muscles active accessory elevators or depressors. That such accessory actions exist, however, is indisputable, but is a consequence of the mechanical relationship of the muscle plane to the center of rotation and is, therefore, a function of the position of the eye or of anatomical variations. The accessory role of the vertical muscles in horizontal rotations can become significant only when the globe has rotated into secondary or tertiary positions. In the latter case, only one vertical mover at a time can exhibit such a component; for example, up and in for the superior rectus, since in the elevated, adducted position the inferior rectus is completely inhibited and the inferior oblique is a pure elevator. Such accessory action is not accompanied by innervational alterations.

The behavior of the horizontal muscles in tertiary positions has been noted to vary;[132] thus the lateral or medial recti may, in some instances, increase in gaze up and out; in others, they may increase in gaze down and out. On the other hand, other studies have shown fair consistency whereby no change in the activity of these muscles is recorded in tertiary plane movements.[109] The vertical muscles in tertiary movements do show alterations; thus the vertical recti appear more active in the abducted state than in the adducted state. The obliques are more active in the adducted state than in the abducted state.[26,31,132] These changes occur in extreme vertical fields of gaze and are not seen within 23° above or below the primary horizontal plane.[109]

The basis for the innervational difference in the vertical muscles between abduction and adduction is not clear. It has been noted that the integrated electromyogram of the horizontal rotators at the peak of their horizontal excursion is higher than at the peak of their oblique excursion. This has been attributed to inhibition.[110] A similar observation was made for the vertical muscles.

SACCADIC MOVEMENT (SEE FIGURE 9). The study of saccadic movements[19,36,106,131] shows that there is an initial large burst in the agonist

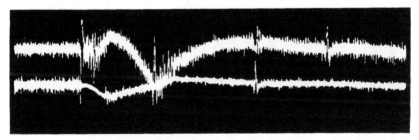

FIGURE 9. ELECTROMYOGRAM IN SACCADIC MOVEMENT

Upper trace, left lateral rectus; *lower trace*, left medial rectus. Primary position with saccades to the left; inhibitions correspond to excitations. No cocontraction.

accompanied by an inhibition of the antagonist. Following the burst, there is a return to the steady state level of innervation characteristic of the new position. The extent of the saccadic burst is proportional to the degree of movement. During a horizontal saccade, there may be brief cocontraction of the vertical muscles. Secondary bursts may be superimposed upon the initial burst and overshoots occur which require compensation. Saccadic movements may achieve very high velocity, reaching 400° per sec. Gliding movements tend to be of smooth character and are to a much less extent accompanied by saccadic bursts. The antagonist in a saccadic movement exhibits an abrupt inhibition with a return of its electric activity at the conclusion of the saccade to the degree requisite in the new position. There are no evidences of braking action of the antagonist, so that the ballistic theory of saccadic ocular movement (wherein the antagonist contracts to halt the action) supported by Alpern and Wolter[4] is not substantiated.[36,106,131] This had been previously demonstrated with optical means by Westheimer,[142] who pointed out the factors involved in orbital resistance to rotation in a detailed analysis of saccadic movement. This is further evidence for the existence of real orbital resistance to movement and indicates that augmentation of contraction in agonists is necessary for maintained rotation.

The electromyographic pattern of saccadic movement is also seen in jerky nystagmus[26] and has been reported in the electromyographic study of eye movement during reading.[19]

POSITION OF REST DURING ANESTHESIA AND SLEEP (SEE FIGURES 10 TO 13)

The tonic activity of the extraocular muscles, which is so characteristic and which falls off to zero or almost zero only in the extreme of gaze out of the field of the muscle, poses questions of considerable physiologic interest. Under what conditions do the ocular muscles achieve electric silence or complete rest? What maintains the tonic activity of the waking state?

SLEEP. It was observed that, during sleep, electric activity of extraocular muscle rapidly fell off to zero,[15] although it was interrupted by short bursts of single units or runs of units during lighter phases, possibly accompanying dream activity.[33] As the subject awakened, the electric activity increased, achieving the normal tonic firing during consciousness.

Simultaneous electro-oculograms demonstrated that the bursts and runs of units were accompanied by small oscillations of the eye, despite the very low amplitude and frequency of the electric activity.[33]

Since the eyes are hardly ever directed so far to one side as to remove innervation from the antagonists, and since the agonists at that point are maximally active, it is obvious that there can be no position of innervational silence during consciousness. It is easy to

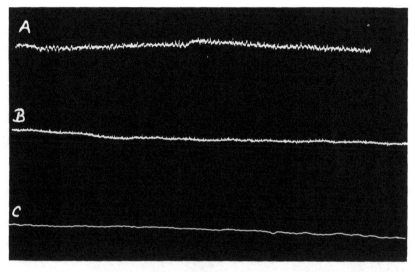

FIGURE 10. ELECTROMYOGRAM OF LATERAL RECTUS; RETROBULBAR PROCAINE
ANESTHESIA

A, before anesthetic was given; B, several minutes after injection; C, complete
electric silence in five minutes.

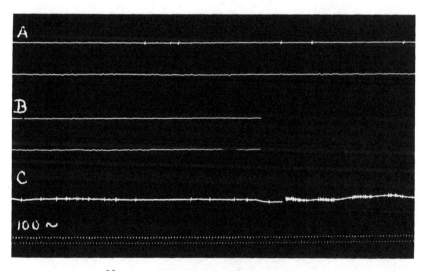

FIGURE 11. ELECTROMYOGRAM OF MEDIAL RECTUS IN SLEEP

A, *upper tracing*, myogram, showing coupled units; *lower tracing*, EOG, showing
no eye movement; B, deep sleep, electric silence; C, light sleep, irregular bursts
and runs of units on awakening, turning into trains and then into normal discharge pattern.

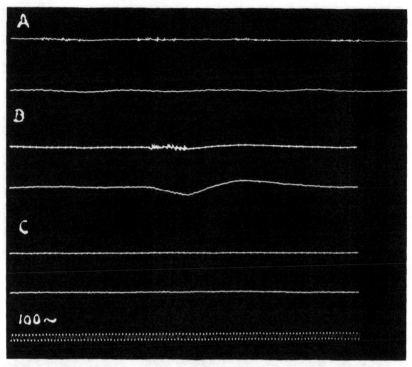

FIGURE 12. ELECTROMYOGRAM OF MEDIAL RECTUS IN SLEEP

A, *upper tracing*, rhythmic trains of potentials; *lower tracing*, undulation of EOG, indicating eye movement with each train; B, *upper*, single unit discharge with one burst eliciting a movement of the globe; *lower*, EOG showing deflection caused by innervation; C, *upper*, single unit discharges; *lower*, EOG, no movement.

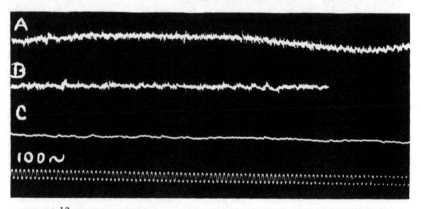

FIGURE 13. ELECTROMYOGRAM OF THE LATERAL RECTUS—GENERAL ANESTHESIA

A, before anesthesia; B, several minutes after thiopental administration; C, surgical plane.

see, therefore, that sleep is the only physiologic process affording the individual relaxation and rest of the extraocular muscles. Since these muscles do not exhibit fatigue, they do not appear to need such innervational rest; however, the central processes subserving fusion do require rest when they are strained through heterophoria. Sleep, therefore, provides relief from asthenopia by removing the fusional burden.

ANESTHESIA. Following local procaine instillation or retrobulbar anesthesia, the action potentials rapidly fall away, achieving electric silence within three to five minutes. The rapid response of the muscle reflects the anatomical-pharmacologic uniformity of extraocular muscle.[33]

During the induction of general anesthesia, roving and vergence movements of the eyes are noted. These movements cease in the surgical plane of anesthesia. During the asphyxial stage, a convergent, depressed position may be assumed. Following induction with thiopental anesthesia, the innervation to the extraocular muscles rapidly decreases, being completely obtunded in the surgical plane. Lightening of the level of anesthesia is accompanied by a recovery of innervation, beginning with small, single units. An increase of the anesthetic level causes a prompt disappearance of the activity. The time interval required for achieving electric silence is only a few minutes. It is theoretically possible, although practically unfeasible, to servo-monitor anesthesia by this activity.

FUNDAMENTAL POSITIONS. The position assumed by the eyes during the surgical plane of anesthesia is not influenced by innervation.[32,33] This position is, therefore, dictated by anatomical-mechanical factors— bony, facial, and muscular—and represents the anatomical position of rest. This is the basic position of the eyes which is modified by numberless innervational factors during consciousness. If this basic position is one of divergence, then a basic stress toward divergence must underlie whatever position the eyes assume in consciousness. It opposes esodeviation and facilitates exodeviation. The frequency of some degree of divergence under surgical anesthesia supports the concept of a basic anatomical divergence to which in exotropia may be added innervational divergence. This basic position also underlies most esotropia and predisposes to the exodeviation of surgical overcorrection or decreased esoinnervation, however induced. The existence of anatomical convergence would, of course, work in the opposite sense. From this starting position, one may obtain the various positions of the eyes (Maddox' vergences) through the outflow of varied innervational sources; namely, the anatomical, tonic, accommodative, and fusional positions and the position influenced by the near or proximal factor.[35] These positions can be suitably separated by control of the proximal, accommodative, fusional, and tonic factors. The tonic factor during consciousness is relatively unsusceptible to influence, but the progress of psychopharmacology may yet produce agents which will control the tonic activity as well.

As will be seen in the section on proprioception, the complete release of the extraocular muscles from the globe in man resulted in a loss of electric activity. The tonic firing was therefore correlated with proprioceptive feedback.[30] Extensive animal studies[40] show that decortication, decerebration, and spinal transection do not *per se* materially reduce tonic firing of extraocular muscle. However, the animal (cat or dog) tends toward a sleeping state with quiescent muscles but is readily aroused by stimuli such as whistling, pinching a paw, or even pulling on the ocular muscle. The depressed activity wells back and can even simulate a stretch reflex. In the cat and dog, release of the extraocular muscle from the globe generally reduced the level of tonic firing, but the central excitatory state appeared more significant. An aroused animal could exhibit high activity in released muscle, while a depressed animal could demonstrate no activity of intact muscle. Although eye movement generally accompanied the heightened discharges, sometimes no movement was seen.

Thus, it has been demonstrated that abundant tonic firing can be maintained by the isolated brainstem. This fact, plus the close correlation of tonic activity with the conscious state and its depression by sleep and anesthesia, strongly implicates the reticular formation and arousal centers in its maintenance. Electric activity of extraocular muscle, however, is demonstrable in comatose patients.[36,121] The "arousal" effect of flicker on the ocular electromyogram[6,80] supports this concept.

LAW OF INNERVATION (SEE FIGURE 14)

The quantity of innervation to the extraocular muscles for a given position of gaze is constant and is the same no matter how the eye arrives at the given position. This holds true for all normal movements of the eye. In vergences, as will be seen later, this is true until the near point of convergence is approximated, at which time cocontraction may occur. It permits the statement of a new law of innervation; namely, "the electric activity of the extraocular muscles parallels the position of the eye." This has been expressed by Breinin[34,39] as follows:

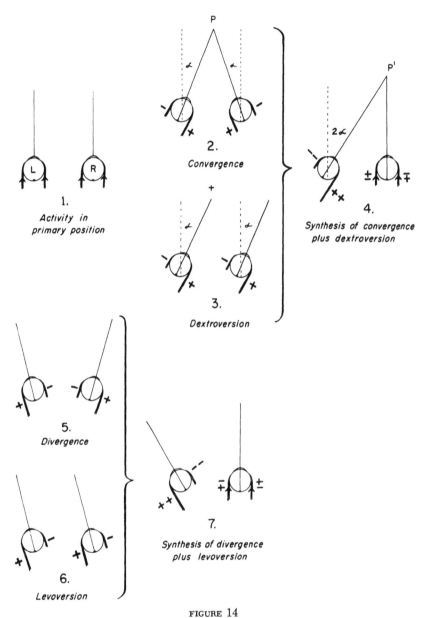

FIGURE 14
See description in text.

All forms of innervation, version, and vergence are centrally integrated, the vector resultant issuing forth in the final common path to the extraocular muscles as a simple reciprocity mechanism. Thus the electric activity of the muscles must vary as the gaze varies; in the absence of movement the electric activity is constant.

Momosse[109] has expressed it as follows:

The quantity of innervation to each extraocular muscle is a function of the position of gaze and the moving velocity of the fixational eye. When the fixation line is in repose it is a function of the position of the eye alone.

Exceptions to this general law of innervation are mechanical limitations of the globe in which the innervation cannot reflect the position of the eye, cocontraction from either normal or abnormal causes, and certain neurogenic or myogenic disturbances. The law may be rephrased in this fashion: Under normal physiologic conditions, if the eye moves, there is an appropriate alteration of innervation; if the innervation alters, the eye moves.

The existence of such a law is disputed by Jampolsky, Tamler, and Marg,[77] who stated that one may not elicit the position of the eye from the innervation. To be sure, the degree of movement cannot be accurately determined but the fact of movement can be determined. The type of movement will be a consequence of the mechanical relationship of the muscle plane to the center of rotation. The evidence adduced by these authors relates essentially to non-physiologic conditions, to conditions not obtaining throughout the range of most normal ocular movement, or to conditions existing only briefly during movement. In this connection, it must be emphasized that *the law of innervation pertains to the steady state existing at the beginning and end of movement.*

VERGENCE (SEE FIGURES 15 TO 21)

MID-LINE. During symmetrical mid-line convergence, the medial recti increase the firing rate, number, and amplitude of motor units. The lateral recti are correspondingly and reciprocally inhibited. When the near point of convergence is reached, there is an increased innervation to the lateral rectus of the diverging eye with a reciprocal inhibition of its medial rectus. As the eye diverges, the innervation parallels the changing position; that is, the lateral rectus increases and the medial rectus decreases in activity. The fixing eye may show little or no change of activity.[21,26]

Several studies[106,107] have shown that, at the breakpoint, following a short latency, the convergence innervation gradually increases with

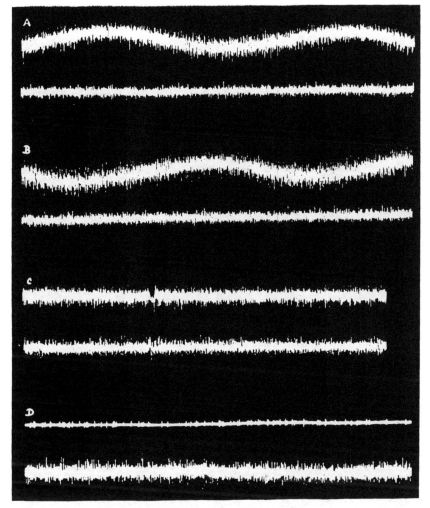

FIGURE 15. APPROXIMATION VERGENCE

Left lateral rectus, *upper trace*; left medial rectus, *lower trace*. Approximation in axis O.S.: A, start; B, end (no change—O.S. stationary) (undulation of upper trace is an artifact). Approximation in axis O.D.: C, start; D, end (change—O.S. converged).

slight change in activity for almost a second. This differs from the burst of saccadic movement and tends to show a more spindle pattern of discharge. More and different units were noted to be present in convergence than in a saccade of equivalent angle. Two kinds of divergence phenomena are described. In one, there is cocontraction of the

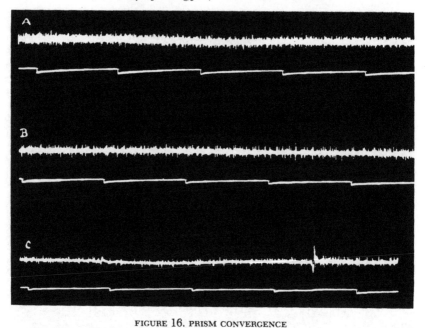

FIGURE 16. PRISM CONVERGENCE

Right lateral rectus, *upper trace*; integrator, *lower trace*. Prisms before O.D.
A, start; B, middle, decreasing; C, end, with divergence.

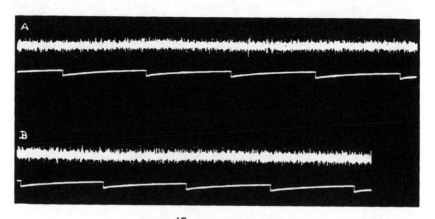

FIGURE 17. PRISM CONVERGENCE

Right lateral rectus, *upper trace*; integrator, *lower trace*. Prisms before O.S.
A, start; B, end (no change).

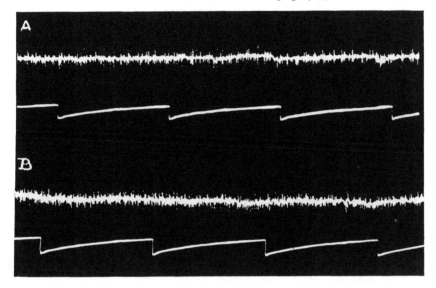

FIGURE 18. ACCOMMODATIVE VERGENCE; MEDIAL RECTUS, LEFT EYE

A, primary position; B, with −1 diopter lens before the right eye (note increased firing and height of integrator discharge). EMG, *above*; integration, *below*.

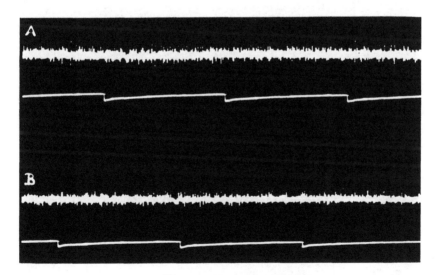

FIGURE 19. ACCOMMODATIVE VERGENCE

Right lateral rectus, *upper trace*; integrator, *lower trace*; −2 sphere before O S. A, before; B, after, decreased as eye converged.

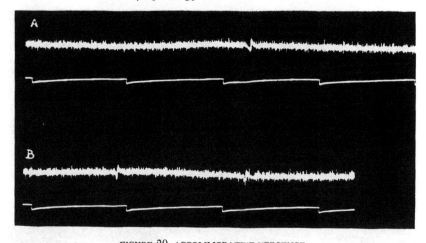

FIGURE 20. ACCOMMODATIVE VERGENCE

Right lateral rectus, *upper trace*; integrator, *lower trace*; —2 sphere before O.D.
A, before; B, after (no change).

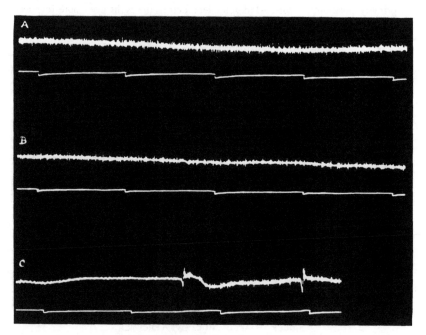

FIGURE 21. APPROXIMATION VERGENCE

Right lateral rectus, *upper trace*; integrator, *lower trace*. Approximation in axis
O.S.: A, start; B, middle (decreases as eye converges); C, end, with divergence.

medial and lateral recti. A saccadic burst in the medial rectus accompanies a spindle pattern of increased activity in the lateral rectus, following which a uniform firing pattern appears. The figure shown, however, suggests that a fine reciprocity may actually be present. The second form of divergence activity is marked by inhibition of the medial rectus with the reappearance of an irregular pattern followed by a steady state of firing. The lateral rectus exhibits a saccade at the time of inhibition of the medial rectus and an irregular pattern reciprocating with the medial rectus until a stable state is reached. Secondary bursts of saccadic movement were also noted during divergence.

Overlapping augmentation of activity in antagonists indicates unequivocally that divergence is active. Such a pattern was noted in a patient with exotropia in an earlier report by Breinin and Moldaver.[26]

Miller[107] reported cocontraction in single units of antagonists during mid-line convergence and found that such activity occurred further away in subjects with a remote near point of convergence. He considers cocontraction a normal variant of divergence.

The increased activity of the lateral rectus may be noted to precede the actual divergence movement by a very brief interval. The increased innervation of the lateral rectus at the breakpoint may also be expressed in a summated potential due to the overlapping discharge of many units.[35]

Nystagmoid innervation of the medial rectus may occur at the breakpoint of convergence and a time lag of 0.2 to 0.3 sec. between the onset of increased breakpoint activity and the actual movement of the eye has been noted.[21] Convergence movement has a much slower velocity than saccadic movement, averaging about 10° per sec. contrasted with several hundred degrees per second for the former.

The fact that saccadic and vergence movements have such different velocities has led to the hypothesis by Alpern and Wolter[4] of a dual innervation to extraocular muscles. Large, somatic, myelinated nerve fibers are considered to innervate muscle fibers subserving saccadic movement. Small, non-myelinated, autonomic nerve fibers are said to innervate the muscle fibers responsible for vergence movement.

This concept was criticized by Brecher and Mitchell,[25] who could demonstrate no effect of sympathetic stimulation upon muscle tension at rest or during movement. Breinin and Perryman[40] could find no effect of topical or systemic epinephrine upon the muscle of cat or man. Attempts at isolation and stimulation of parasympathetic nerves to the extraocular muscles are in progress.

It is clear that a number of patterns of activity may be observed in antagonistic muscles during mid-line convergence at or near the breakpoint. It is probable that such variations reflect an interplay of fusional effort to counteract the divergence tendency. It is also clear from all the studies presented that divergence is an active phenomenon which cannot be construed as being due solely to the relaxation of the medial rectus with an accompanying passive, elastic, musculo-skeletal divergence stress.[21,26,107] The existence of active divergence lends strength to the concept of an independent divergence function. The source of such innervation remains unknown but clearly reflects a central, independent process. The active divergence of intermittent exotropia supports the above conclusions.

It is of interest that following a maximal symmetrical mid-line convergence, upon carrying the gaze to the side, the agonist medial rectus exhibits an increase in its potentials with accompanying inhibition of its antagonist lateral rectus. The limitation of convergence, therefore, is not due to exhaustion of the power of the medial rectus, but is a central phenomenon.

The greater adduction of the eye in conjugate gaze has been attributed to the additional effect of the vertical recti acting as active accessory adductors. The vertical recti, however, maintain their usual tonic innervational level. Whatever accessory role the vertical recti exert in adduction is due solely to the mechanical relation of their muscle planes to the center of rotation. The innervational role must be ascribed to the agonist in the movement and not to the auxiliary muscles.[31]

In convergence below the horizontal plane, the inferior rectus is active; its level of discharge, however, is related not to convergence but to the degree of depression of the globe. Since intorsion is said to occur with convergence and not extortion, its activity as an extorter must be overcome, presumably by the medial rectus acting as an intorter. This may be a function of the vertical level of convergence.

ASYMMETRIC. Because of the great relevance of the vergence mechanisms to the problem of strabismus, studies of asymmetric vergence have been of particular interest. When a fixation object is smoothly and gradually approximated along the fixation axis of one eye, the eye remains stationary. The other eye must make a large excursion to maintain fixation; if it is covered, it still moves in response to accommodative vergence.

Electromyography reveals that the moving eye demonstrates large alterations in the activity of its horizontal muscles with the medial rectus increasing and the lateral rectus decreasing. However, in the stationary eye there is no change of activity in the horizontal muscles for at least 10–16 or more meter angles of asymmetric convergence.[21,27,35,107,109]

At or near the breakpoint, simultaneous augmentation of medial and lateral rectus muscles may occur.[107,129] Such cocontraction is not encountered during most of the physiologic range of vergence. In monocular asymmetric vergence, jump or smooth, there is no movement of the fixing eye and no alteration of activity of the horizontal muscles.

Breinin,[27,35] Blodi,[21] and Momosse[109] have reported similar observations. Tamler, Jampolsky, and Marg,[129] on the other hand, have denied that the non-moving eye shows no alteration and maintain that cocontraction always occurs. Alpern[5] stated that in smooth asymmetric vergence no change would be expected in the non-moving eye. Miller[107] described both responses depending upon the type of experiment. In smooth vergence his findings supported the concept of a central integrating mechanism. Breinin has modified Hering's explanation of the phenomenon, stating it must be an example of central integration within the brain of the innervations of vergence and version, such that the convergence innervation in the stationary eye is neutralized by an opposing version innervation. The moving eye, however, gets a double dose of innervation of vergence plus version in the same direction.[27,35] In the non-moving eye, the algebraic summation of excitations and inhibitions of the two forms of innervation results in the same level of activity as existed previously in the primary position. It therefore shows no alteration of activity of its horizontal recti. Although Hering[69] believed the neutralization occurred peripherally in the form of a cocontraction of the horizontal muscles of the non-moving eye, this has been shown not to occur throughout the physiologic range of movement.

The authors of the alternative viewpoint have stacked the cards in favor of their hypothesis by eliciting the phenomenon at the near point. The occurrence of cocontraction can be explained by the fact that the central integrating mechanism may break down at the near point with a consequent spilling over of opposing innervation into the final common path. The fact that a physiologic process can have a limiting point is not remarkable. Tamler, Jampolsky, and Marg maintain that Hering's law has been misinterpreted. There is no misinterpretation involved; there is a question solely of the locus of neutralization of opposing innervations which, according to Hering, occurs peripherally and which, according to Breinin, occurs centrally.

Numbers of inconsistencies have been pointed out in the data of

Tamler, Jampolsky, and Marg[5,22,120] (*vide supra*). Furthermore, they also noted that in monocular approximation, despite the accommodative vergence being exerted, no alteration occurred in the non-moving eye. This is a complete negation of their own position.

The optical studies of Westheimer and Mitchell[143] and the electrooculographic studies of Alpern and Wolter[4] demonstrated the fractionation of rapid, binocular asymmetric convergence into a conjugate movement followed by a convergence back to achieve fixation. Alpern and Ellen[3] reported similarly that both eyes moved with binocular, rapid asymmetric convergence, but when fixation was carried out monocularly no movement of the fixing eye occurred. These results are based upon the experimental technique. Binocular jump vergence induced by either prisms or a sudden shifting of gaze from distance to near fixation is accompanied by a gross movement of both eyes which can readily be seen. This movement is identical with that which often occurs in the intermittent exotrope upon uncovering a deviated dominant eye, although the movement is damped when uncovering a non-dominant eye. If, however, the experiment is conducted with gradual, smooth approximation of a test object along the fixation axis of the one eye, or if gradual vergence is obtained by means of a rotary prism or haploscope, then central integration of the opposing innervations is carried out so that no movement or electric alteration occurs in the non-moving eye. When the near point of convergence is reached, cocontraction at times may occur. The abrupt discontinuity of fixation which occurs with the sudden interposition of a prism, sudden change from distance to near fixation, or by uncovering a deviated eye will induce a breakdown of the central integrating mechanism. This may also occur at the near point of vergence, but these data do not vitiate the fundamental rule of constancy of innervation in a non-moving eye. Indeed, following such jump movements when the deviated eye returns to fix, the same steady state of innervation that existed prior to the movement and which is characteristic for that position of the eye is demonstrated.

It is possible but not probable that the failure to record innervational alteration of the non-moving eye is due to inadequate sampling of the entire muscle. It is also unlikely that vergence movements are independent of Hering's law. The differences between the binocular and monocular experiment of asymmetric convergence may relate to the influence of visual factors (retinal feedback) in disrupting the central integrating apparatus.

One suggested explanation[3] of these experiments implicated a dual innervation consisting of somatic version and autonomic vergence. The effect of the former was considered to outweigh the latter. This appears improbable because whether the innervation is somatic or autonomic in the non-moving eye, the end result must be cocontraction. This does not occur within 16-M. angles of convergence. Therefore, the innervations must have neutralized one another at a higher level than the final common path, and this can only reflect the central integrating mechanism. It is, furthermore, difficult to conceive of a mechanism capable of simultaneously adjusting somatic and autonomic innervation in this fashion. A peripheral adjustment of opposing innervations always requires cocontraction and such cocontraction, even in the cases which exhibit dual movements, is not apparent when the eye has regained fixation. Therefore, the validity of Hering's law of distributed innervation throughout the physiologic range of binocular movements is reaffirmed with the addition that the locus of adjustment of opposing innervations must be central.

The application of this concept of opposing innervations carries through to strabismus in which the deviations must be deemed disturbances not simply of vergence but of combined vergence and version in the interest of maintaining fixation in one eye. The studies in asymmetric vergence further support the law of innervation; namely, if the innervation does not alter, the eye does not move, and when the eye moves, the innervation alters, within physiological limits.

LENS OR PRISM INDUCED. The effect of a lens in augmenting or inhibiting accommodative vergence can be readily evaluated. Minus lenses elicit increasing amounts of accommodative vergence and hence increased levels of firing in the medial rectus of a non-fixing eye. This activity does not appear in the medial rectus of the fixing eye, since fixation precludes any change of innervation. When both eyes fix, neither shows any change, since accommodative convergence is negated by fusional divergence. The same phenomena are noted when prisms or haploscopes are employed. The moving eye will always exhibit the appropriate alteration of innervation as its accommodative or fusional vergence is altered. The stationary eye shows no change in accordance with the corrective, neutralizing innervation of the opposite version mediated by the central integrating apparatus.[31,32,35]

Studies on the haploscope show that from the dissociated position fusional divergence is accompanied by increased activity in the lateral rectus of the diverging eye.[35] Such activity is difficult to demonstrate because of the small amplitudes of fusional divergence which come close to the limits of sensitivity of the technique.

An interesting corollary of the studies with lenses and prisms is that fusional training is essentially a central process and cannot result in increased power of muscles.

OCULAR MUSCLE PROPRIOCEPTION (SEE FIGURES 22 TO 24)

Although Sherrington believed that the extraocular muscles possess a proprioceptive mechanism giving rise to position sense,[126] all the experimental studies that have been done in the last several decades have tended to disprove this notion.[44,53,101,102,119] The information derived from vision and the innervational urge are considered the

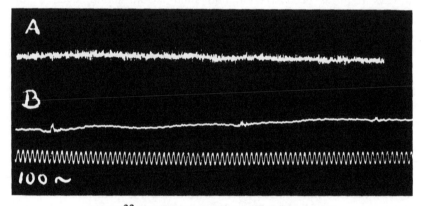

FIGURE 22. ELECTROMYOGRAM OF A RECTUS MUSCLE

A, before severance of tendon; B, after severance of tendon (note decreased activity). Amplitude of time signal, 100 μv.

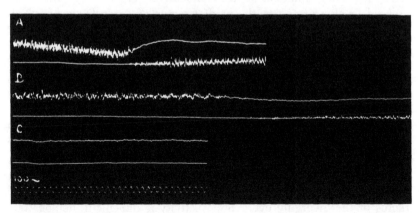

FIGURE 23. ELECTROMYOGRAM OF MEDIAL AND LATERAL RECTUS AFTER ENUCLEATION

A, reciprocal innervation rapid; B, reciprocal innervation slow; C, primary position, no activity. Amplitude of time signal, 100 μv.

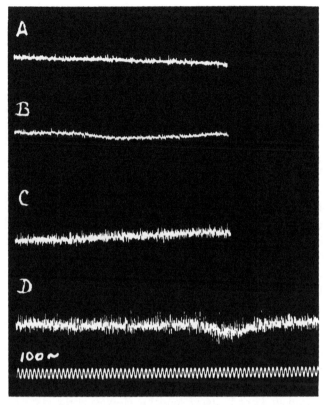

FIGURE 24. ELECTROMYOGRAM OF PARETIC LATERAL RECTUS
A, primary position, low amplitude and frequency; B, abduction, low activity; C, adduction, anomalously increased innervation; D, passive adduction, even greater anomalous activity. Amplitude of time signal, 100 μv.

adequate basis of our awareness or lack of awareness of eye position. That the extraocular muscles should lack a mechanism for the recording of muscle tension, however, would place them so far apart from other skeletal muscle as to arouse wonder and doubt that they should be so distinguished.[30] That they do have anatomical and pharmacologic peculiarities, however, has been long appreciated. The extraocular muscles have been noted to contain an abundance of unusual nerve endings, as well as nerve fibers of two distinct types: large myelinated fibers and small non-myelinated fibers. The hypothetical role of these fibers has been previously discussed.

For many years the existence of muscle spindles in extraocular muscle was denied. However, the pioneer studies of Cooper and co-workers[48,49,50,52] have abundantly confirmed their existence. These authors have recorded typical stretch discharges in afferent fibers coursing in the third, fourth, and sixth nerves, via the fifth nerve, and in the brainstem, providing clear neurophysiologic evidence for the existence of a tension recording apparatus in extraocular muscles.[50] Spindles have been found in some animals and not others. They have not been seen in the rabbit, dog, cat, or monkey, but are abundantly present in the goat, higher apes, and man.[45,48,50] These spindles are somewhat different from those found in the peripheral musculature and exhibit a number of intrafusal fibers. Despite the absence of spindles, stretch of the cat and monkey extraocular muscle produced proprioceptive discharges.[52] The number of proprioceptors in the extraocular muscles has been found to be of the same magnitude as that in the lumbrical muscles of the hands, and they are usually located in the proximal third of the muscle.[48]

Anatomical and electrophysiologic evidence indicates that branches of the trigeminal are distributed to the extraocular muscles and mainly carry impulses from the muscle spindles. The cell bodies for these proprioceptive fibers are considered by many to lie within the mesencephalic root of the trigeminal nerve.

The muscle spindles described by Cooper and Daniel in 1949 have been criticized, however, as inadequate to subserve a proprioceptive position sense, a function which would actually be disadvantageous to the organism (Lord Charnwood[44]). However, the data from peripheral proprioceptors of muscle and tendon do not reach consciousness but are integrated in the cerebellum.

The question of proprioception in the extraocular muscles is an old one. Early studies concerning nystagmus brought up the question of whether the fast phase was induced by stretch of the muscle during the slow phase. Bartels[9] theorized that such was the case. De Kleyn[53] paralyzed the proprioceptive endings with procaine in the decerebrate rabbit in an attempt to selectively paralyze sensory before motor endings. This resulted only in the eventual paralysis of the muscle. Caloric stimulation of the labyrinths produced typical contractions and relaxations with no disturbance attributable to loss of proprioception. This was considered to disprove a muscular origin of the rapid phase.

McIntyre[102] studied the nerves to the extraocular muscles of cats under light ether narcosis. A tonic discharge was present in all of the nerves examined. This discharge diminished or disappeared in deep anesthesia. Cutting the motor nerve to a muscle did not seem to alter the discharge in the central end. Cutting all of the motor nerves to the extraocular muscles did not alter neural nystagmus patterns, indicating their central origin. McIntyre concluded that proprioceptive endings in the extraocular muscle do not seem essential for the maintenance of their tonus or activity.

Working with decerebrate cats, McCouch and Adler[101] were unable to alter tension or nystagmus patterns by stretch of the extraocular muscles. They confirmed the work of Hoffmann,[71] who reported the absence of the stretch reflex in the extraocular muscle of the cat. All previous experimental data also indicated that stretch reflexes in extraocular muscle could not be elicited.

Since the extraocular muscles are not extensor muscles in which phasic and static stretch reflexes are best obtained, it would not be expected that tendon jerk responses should occur.

In a study by Breinin[30] of the electromyography of the extraocular muscles during enucleation procedures, local anesthesia, light enough to permit ocular movements, was employed. Considerable pre-anesthetic sedation was required. When the muscles were cut away from their connection to the globe, the level of firing decreased. Following complete retraction of the muscles into the equilibrium position, obtained by cutting away all supporting fascia, the activity ceased. They now resembled peripheral skeletal muscle at rest. On attempted gaze to the side, however, they promptly fired and demonstrated a reciprocity pattern. This pattern differed from that obtained prior to the release of the muscles in that the gradation of the reciprocity mechanism appeared altered. The activity of the agonist commenced abruptly with abrupt inhibition in the antagonist, whereas, previously, the activity in both had overlapped.

The attempt to augment motor discharge in a retracted muscle above the level found just prior to cutting the tendon by means of stretching was unsuccessful. No inhibiting effect on the antagonist was noted from stretch of the agonist. In this study, the patient's good eye was directed straight forward. It was concluded that retraction of the free muscle disburdens a spindle mechanism which ceases its discharge and thus inhibits motor unit firing. The alterations in reciprocal innervation were also attributed to the loss of an afferent mechanism maintaining the normal level and gradation of firing. These data were considered to support the concept of a proprioceptive tension recording mechanism in extraocular muscle of man. It appeared clear that phasic stretch (tendon jerk) did not occur, but that a basic static stretch mechanism which could not be augmented beyond a limiting point was present.

The tonic firing of the primary position was attributed to a spindle mechanism activating the muscles through a certain amount of stretch. Recent animal experimentation[40] has confirmed the depression of activity in fully released muscle and implicated the reticular formation and "arousal" in its genesis (*vide infra*).

In a study of stretch effects in human extraocular muscle by Sears, Teasdall, and Stone,[122] no alteration was obtained in the firing pattern of a muscle before and after severance of its tendon from the globe, although the authors state that they did not obtain complete retraction of the muscle during enucleation procedures. They, too, did not encounter any stretch reflex or augmentation of innervation by stretch of any muscle in the primary position. During active agonist contraction, however, stretch of the agonist itself, its antagonist, or yoke muscle induced inhibitory responses in the agonist. The authors concluded that there are receptors in extraocular muscle which are sensitive to stretch. It is not clear why these effects were only noted in gaze movements and not in the primary position. Furthermore, their finding of inhibitory responses through forced ductions is contrary to the experience of others.

Bjork[18] had shown that passive movements of the eye did not alter the pattern of electric activity in the extraocular muscles and that the innervation accorded with the innervational urge. This was confirmed by Breinin and Moldaver.[26]

The arousal concept of activation of the extraocular muscles accords well with what is known of the response of these muscles in man to anesthesia, sleep,[33] and flickering light.[80] It must be concluded, therefore, that the existence of proprioceptive end organs in human extraocular muscle has been demonstrated, but the function of such end organs cannot be stated with certainty.

The concept of anomalous innervation[30] deserves mention in this connection. This was encountered in a small percentage of paretic muscles wherein the muscle augmented its discharge away from its field of action. In abducens palsy, the lateral rectus, which may have shown very little activity into its field, exhibited more marked activity away from its field and thus behaved as though it were its own antagonist. In some instances, passive rotation of the globe also elicited an abundant firing pattern away from the field of the muscle. During nystagmus, both muscles recruited in the same direction. This bizarre activity was attributed to a stretch mechanism made manifest by the paresis.

The concept of anomalous innervation has been criticized as a normal electromyographic variation or as being due to artifactual activity.[77] The existence of activity increasing in opposite directions when recording from the overlapping area of the inferior rectus and inferior oblique is an example cited. This criticism has merit. There is no doubt that recording at the overlapped site of inferior rectus and inferior oblique could give rise to the picture of anomalous innervation. This was not the case in the patients described by Breinin. In an investigation of some abducens palsies that exhibited anomalous innervation, it could be seen that deep electrode probing in the paretic lateral rectus muscle to elicit activity could result in sampling the area around the insertion of the inferior oblique, with consequent pickup from that muscle. Such activity, at times, was observed to increase in adduction as the electrode and muscle mass approximated to one another, while the activity regressed in abduction as the electrode and muscle mass separated. This is a more likely source of confusion and explains why such activity was not encountered in normal muscles.

The critical differentiation was made by the fact that in elevation of the eye the activity increased more than in other directions of gaze and was inhibited in gaze down. Such an inferior oblique confusion pattern could readily be mistaken as anomalous innervation. This would also be true for passive rotations which could plunge the electrode deeper toward the inferior oblique at that site.

Anomalous innervation is, of course, a characteristic of aberrant regeneration in third nerve palsies. There can be no doubt that this is a legitimate pattern reflecting a discrete, reproducible electric disturbance. When recording from the inferior oblique at its origin, there can be no question of any interference from the inferior rectus. This has never been observed and the anomalous pattern is readily detectable in that site. The medial rectus also gives rise to an anomalous pattern in the aberrant regeneration syndrome. Although this usually decreases in abduction, it may at times increase if an element of elevation or depression occurs. In some instances, anomalous activity may be attributable to unusual irritability. Stretching the muscle fibers with the electrode may produce discharge bursts due to irritation of the fibers. Such bursts are similar to those seen during insertion of an electrode. It should be noted that in normal muscle single units have been reported which increase their firing rate out of the field of action.[86,88]

The concept of anomalous innervation based upon a stretch mechanism, therefore, is rightfully criticized, since many factors may be of importance in its genesis. Nevertheless, it cannot be discarded since some instances do not conform with any other known causative factors.

Part of the general problem of proprioception lies in the difficulty of obtaining the experimental data in man and in the extreme importance of the level and type of anesthesia and sedation, which can grossly alter the findings.[40] It cannot be stated that we have any clear understanding of these mechanisms, or, indeed, of the basic data involved.

NYSTAGMUS (SEE FIGURE 25)

Much of the early investigation of the extraocular muscles was concerned with the problem of nystagmus.[53,70,71,81,82,94,101,102,115,118,119] The question of extraocular muscle proprioception entered largely into the theoretical discussion of the causation of the fast and slow phases. It is generally accepted that the control of the rhythm of nystagmus is

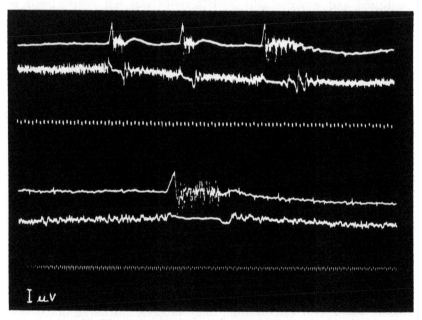

FIGURE 25. CALORIC NYSTAGMUS (COLD WATER IN RIGHT EAR)

Upper, left lateral rectus; *lower*, right lateral rectus. Time, 100 cycles. In upper tracings extremely rapid nystagmus episodes occurred. Note reciprocal relationship between these contralateral antagonists. Base line showed absence of activity in the left lateral rectus corresponded to complete silence of the right lateral rectus, owing to gaze being directed to the right; a sudden burst of marked activity in the left lateral rectus corresponded to complete silence of the right lateral rectus. One nystagmus episode is recorded from the same muscle at fast speed (time, 100 cycles).

central and that the effector organ does not alter the pattern, so that proprioception can play no part in its genesis. This may not be altogether true of man where release of muscles from the globe modified the nystagmus timing and abolished the tonic outflow. It is unlikely that electrode position changes were responsible for these alterations.

The reciprocity mechanism,[124,125,127] first elucidated by Sherrington, was later shown by many others during nystagmus investigations.[53,70,71,94,101,102] In 1935, Lorente de Nó showed that as the speed of nystagmus in rabbits increased, more and more deviation from pure reciprocity occurred. He attributed the differences to time delay circuits. He considered that reciprocal innervation could not be due to a fixed anatomical mechanism. Nystagmus with cocontraction, however, occurred only after lesions of the nervous system. He noted that nystagmus innervation of eye muscles was essentially like spinal muscles in reflex or voluntary activity.

Most studies have emphasized the purity of nystagmus reciprocity. This usual purity may be degraded by narcosis.

The postulated inhibitory effects of stretch[122] do not seem operative during nystagmus, since no alterations of pattern or rhythm were demonstrated in many earlier studies of stretch of extraocular muscles. Furthermore, such stretch did not alter the firing pattern of the nerves to the extraocular muscles.[101,102]

The slow phase of nystagmus is characterized by a slowly increasing rate of discharge and recruitment of motor units in the agonist. At the same time, there is a reciprocal decrease in activity of the antagonist. During the fast phase, there is a sudden burst of activity within the agonist and a reciprocal abrupt inhibition of the antagonist. It is possible that cocontraction in auxiliary muscles may occur during the fast phase. This is not seen during the slow phase. Vertical nystagmus shows a similar picture. The foregoing is the description of jerky nystagmus as exemplified in opticokinetic and vestibular nystagmus.[19,26] Pendular nystagmus, on the other hand, shows a spindle pattern of innervation with a gradually increasing and then decreasing firing pattern in the agonist and a reciprocal pattern in the antagonist.[36] The abrupt bursts of jerky nystagmus are not seen. The jerky pattern of nystagmus is also exemplified by saccadic movement during fixation shifts and reading, and in the small jerks occurring during maintained fixation. The combination of electro-oculography with electromyography permits a detailed analysis of both the innervation to the extraocular muscles and the consequent movement of the globe.[19,29,33]

The electric activity in muscle precedes the movement. The initial burst in the agonist in saccadic movement and in nystagmus bears a relation to the extent of the movement, the larger movements requiring longer bursts. The speed of the slow phase is proportional to the extent of the movement.

The recruitment of units is asynchronous in the burst, although the almost simultaneous discharge results in integration of voltage. To some extent this can be separated by fast sweeps.

The functional modification of extraocular muscle enabling extreme rapidity of action is exemplified by the extraordinarily high rates of ocular movement encountered in nystagmus.[26,94]

ABNORMAL ELECTRIC PATTERNS

The principal role of general electromyography has been to elucidate qualitative differences between normal and abnormal muscle. Electromyography is of prime importance in establishing the diagnosis of lower motor neuron disturbances. These disturbances are reflected by alterations of the electric wave form, amplitude, and frequency and the pattern of electric firing.

The following studies will demonstrate that extraocular and peripheral skeletal muscle respond similarly to disease.

NEUROGENIC PALSY (SEE FIGURE 26). Neurogenic paresis of moderate to severe degree is indicated by irregular or sparse recruitment, poorly sustained discharge, and loss of the interference pattern characteristically seen on effort.[17,29] There may be a greater incidence of single

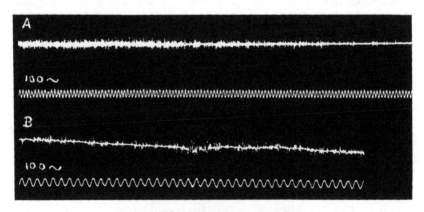

FIGURE 26. PARETIC MEDIAL RECTUS

A, good activity but poorly sustained; B, irregular firing, one nystagmus burst. The amplitude of the time signal is 100 μv. in both traces.

unit discharges in the field of action of a muscle and denervation fibrillations may be encountered. In severe paresis of extraocular muscle, the motor units are usually of decreased amplitude. In general, there is a decreased density of potentials.

The electromyographic pattern of mild palsies is indistinguishable from the normal, since there is a sufficient reserve of units to establish an interference pattern.[17] Units may fire at increased frequencies in palsies, apparently attempting to compensate for the muscle weakness.

In extraocular muscle it is rare to find electric silence. Even in complete clinical palsies one usually encounters some unit activity, often of surprising degree. Conduction block, however, does occur and is attended by complete electric silence.[34]

The cardinal sign of denervation is fibrillation, the minute discharge of single muscle fiber potentials which occur spontaneously without relation to volition.[54,55] Slow, positive waves of denervation have also been described. Characteristic fibrillations have been noted in extraocular muscle palsies,[17,29] although their occurrence is rarely recognized. Caution is necessary in the interpretation of ocular muscle potentials, since small, single motor units bear a very close resemblance to fibrillations. In the absence of volitional potentials, there is no difficulty in classifying fibrillation, but where volition is present the diagnosis must be restricted to the spontaneous potentials which occur when the gaze is directed out of the field of the affected muscle and which evidence no volitional increase in frequency. The finding of denervation phenomena indicates a protracted recovery, if any, and they may persist until reinnervation or fibrosis and atrophy occur.

Polyphasic units are very infrequently encountered in normal extraocular muscles but do occur in abnormal conditions. They are found in paretic peripheral skeletal muscle and are thought to be due to temporal or spatial dispersion of the nerve action current, resulting in asynchronous discharge of the many muscle fibers of a unit. Their relative rarity in extraocular muscle reflects its anatomical uniformity and low innervation ratio. Coupled or grouped firing of units in extraocular muscle may occur. This consists of the synchronized activation of a few motor units and has been attributed in peripheral muscle to a lack of proprioceptive impulses. Whether this is the case in the extraocular muscles is unknown.

Reinnervation units are potentials of large amplitude and long duration, presumably due to the reinnervation of many muscle fibers with a single axon, exceeding the normal innervation ratio. Such units have been reported in third and sixth nerve lesions.[78] They are particularly characteristic of the syndrome of aberrant regeneration.[29,34]

Triphasic wave forms may normally be encountered owing to the effects of volume conduction. These source-sink-source waves occur when the electrode is located at the mid-point in volume.

It must be re-emphasized that the electromyographic pattern of mild palsies is indistinguishable from the normal because of the presence of adequate reserve units which create an interference pattern on effort. Except in complete conduction block or total denervation, some volitional discharge is nearly always present in the paretic muscle.

PSEUDOPARESIS (SEE FIGURE 27). The occurrence of apparent paresis due to anomalies or disturbances of a non-innervational nature is not infrequent. In general, this type of disorder can be recognized by the limited motility shown in the forced duction test. Electromyography

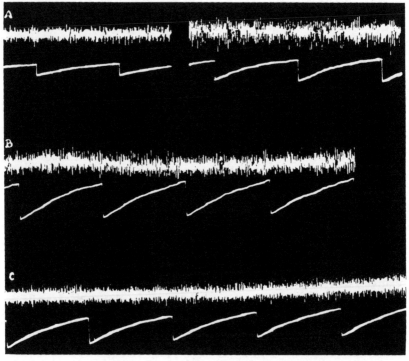

FIGURE 27. ELECTROMYOGRAM IN TENDON SHEATH SYNDROME (O.D.)

Upper trace, inferior oblique; *lower trace*, integrator. A, right inferior oblique: *left*, gaze up and out; *right*, gaze up and in; B, left inferior oblique, gaze up and in; C, left inferior oblique, gaze up and out. Good activity of pseudoparetic
R.I.O.

has proved useful in establishing whether or not an apparently paretic muscle has a normal innervation.[29] For example, one patient with a large esotropia demonstrated a normal electric activity of the lateral rectus despite complete inability to abduct the globe. At surgery, numerous facial bands around the medial rectus were found, limiting abduction. Severance of these bands permitted good abduction of the globe.

The superior oblique sheath syndrome of Brown provides another example of pseudoparesis. The apparently totally paretic inferior oblique muscle can be shown in most cases to fire normally or almost normally. Despite this, there is total inability to elevate the globe. Forced ductions reveal limitation of elevation. Electromyography is helpful in establishing the prognosis.[17,34]

In some cases with abundant electric activity, surgery to the superior oblique has been followed by good rotation into the upper field. In one instance, an overaction of the previously apparently paretic muscle was obtained. Not all cases respond in this fashion, however, and it is likely that other limiting factors are present, the nature of which is not apparent.

Cases of blowout fracture of the orbit have been studied electromyographically.[41] This technique may be of considerable aid to the surgeon in determining prognosis. Where the electric activity of apparently paretic muscles is normal, it is likely that the limitation of rotation is due to mechanical incarceration of the muscles (inferior rectus, inferior oblique) in the fracture line. Where the electric activity of these muscles is defective, damage to the nerve is probable. A combination of both factors may be present. These are practical observations of considerable value and readily obtainable.

PRIMARY AND SECONDARY DEVIATION (SEE FIGURE 28). Hering's law of distributed innervation has been illustrated electromyographically by the increased innervation of secondary deviation and upshoot.[27]

An illustration of this law by Tamler, Jampolsky, and Marg[133] involved the procainization of the medial rectus of the left eye. Saccades of the right eye demonstrated an increased level of activity in the right lateral rectus following the induced paralysis of the left medial rectus. This is a specious demonstration since gross movements are involved, fixation with the paretic eye is not achieved, and the activity is not compared in the same reference position.

OVERACTION. Although underactions of the extraocular muscle may be readily demonstrated electromyographically when they are moderate or severe, overaction is much more difficult to establish. Multiple

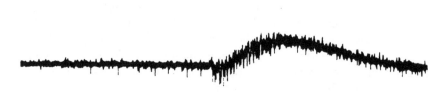

100
I μV

FIGURE 28. LEFT INFERIOR OBLIQUE IN A PATIENT WITH PARETIC RIGHT SUPERIOR
RECTUS

Upper left, good eye fixing in primary position—primary deviation; *upper right,*
paretic eye fixing in primary position—secondary deviation; *lower,* upshoot of
inferior oblique.

electrode insertions are necessary to define either under- or over-action,
but when the activity is clearly much higher than normal, one may
consider the possibility of overactivity. Such overactivity has been
seen in what was clinically spastic esotropia.[36] The finding of overaction does not establish a diagnosis of spasm, but the presence in
clinically spastic muscles of a very high activity appears significant.
For this reason, the exception[77] taken to this concept is considered
without basis.

ABNORMAL NYSTAGMUS. The clear-cut reciprocity patterns of opticokinetic nystagmus have already been described. Muscle paretic
nystagmus is readily demonstrable and shows a similar reciprocity
mechanism. Muscle paretic nystagmus can be readily produced in
normal individuals following prolonged recording and is increased
with multiple needle insertions.

RETRACTORY AND CONVERGENCE NYSTAGMUS (SEE FIGURE 29). A patient
with brain tumor revealed a loss of voluntary vertical gaze associated
with retractory and convergence nystagmus.[29] Electromyograms of the

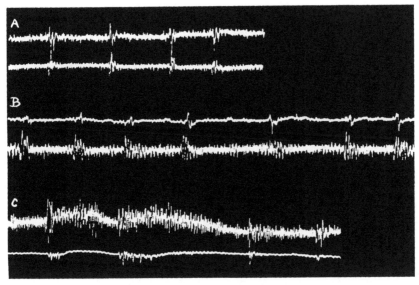

FIGURE 29. RETRACTORY AND CONVERGENCE NYSTAGMUS, RIGHT EYE
Simultaneous recruitment; lateral rectus, *above*; medial rectus, *below*. A, primary
position: retractory nystagmus; B, convergence nystagmus; C, abduction.

horizontal recti revealed almost simultaneous discharge of the antagonists with resultant retraction of the globe. The usual pure reciprocity relationship of nystagmus was completely absent and cocontraction was evident. This was attributed to a supranuclear disturbance
of the reciprocity mechanism. The pattern in retractory and convergence nystagmus was similar. With the eyes convergent, convergence nystagmus was evident. With the eyes in the primary position or in abduction, retractory nystagmus was evident. The occurrence
of such simultaneous innervations has been criticized as possibly due
to an artifact originating in the eyelids.[77] To be sure, electromyograms
obtained during active eye movement must always be viewed with
caution, and the argument is supported by the experimental demonstration of simultaneous electric activity due to lid movement superimposed upon several normal muscle traces. The possibility of such
confusion exists but is most unlikely in the case cited.

Patients should be studied with due precautions taken to obviate
the possibility of such artifacts.

DIABETIC NEUROPATHY. Extraocular muscle palsies associated with
diabetes have been infrequently recognized. They are characterized

by sudden onset, often with severe pain. In most cases the condition clears within six weeks, leaving no *sequelae*. Denervation and aberrant regeneration are rare following such lesions.

Electromyography[34] in a number of such patients showed that the extraocular muscles exhibited either minute potentials or none at all, the trace being almost electrically silent. The appearance was suggestive of the tourniquet-type paralyses in which conduction block prevents the discharge of muscle fibers. Upon recovery of functional activity the electric patterns were restored to normal.

It has been pointed out that electric silence in the extraocular muscles is distinctly unusual. Denervation phenomena usually begin within two weeks following the onset of the lesion.

In diabetic neuropathy, electric silence may persist for more than two weeks. In sudden palsies with absence of electric activity, one should consider the possibility of diabetes. It is probable that electric silence is associated with nerve trunk lesions rather than with nuclear lesions. In one proven case of diabetic neuropathy which came for autopsy, there was a focal inflammation within the trunk of the third nerve.[58] Possibly ischemia is responsible for a transient demyelination of the nerve with consequent conduction block. With the subsidence of the pathological process, resumption of activity occurs. It is of interest that the diabetes in such cases may be of a very latent nature requiring careful diagnostic studies for its demonstration.

Conductive block resulting from various compression lesions may occur within the orbit or cranium, producing complete palsy and loss of innervation. They have a more protracted course and may eventually denervate.

ABERRANT REGENERATION (MISDIRECTION SYNDROME) (SEE FIGURE 30). Following third nerve lesions, in particular those associated with cerebral aneurysms, there may be a total palsy of the muscles innervated by the oculomotor nerve. There ensues a period in which fibrillation may be encountered. Then a reinnervation process begins in which volitional activity returns but with many reinnervation-type units. Clinically, this entity is characterized by elevation of the lid and adduction whenever a movement is attempted into the field of the third nerve complex of muscles. Miosis may also occur. The condition remains permanently.

From experimental lesions in the monkey, Bender and Fulton[11] concluded that random misdirection from a regenerating third nerve results in fibers for all components of the nerve being distributed to all the muscles innervated. On any attempted movement except ab-

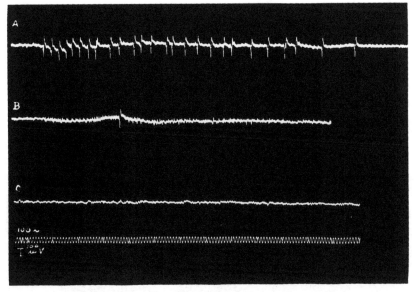

FIGURE 30. LEVATOR SHOWING ABERRANT REGENERATION
A, gaze down; B, gaze in; C, gaze up.

duction, the antagonistic vertical muscles are simultaneously innervated and thus neutralize each other; whereas, the unopposed medial
rectus, levator, and sphincter pupillae account for the adduction of
the globe, retraction of the lid, and miosis respectively. Incomplete
forms of this syndrome occur, particularly with respect to the intraocular muscle.

In every case studied with electromyography,[29,34] the innervation
of the extraocular muscles confirmed the hypothesis of Bender and
Fulton.[11] Thus, the levator fired large units on gaze down, sometimes
with greater activity than on gaze up. It also fired on adduction of
the globe. The superior and inferior vertical muscles fired both into
and out of their field of action, an example of true anomalous innervation.

This entity cannot possibly be considered as artifactual and due to
the overlapping of the recording area of muscles, such as the inferior
rectus and inferior oblique, since it occurs with muscles in which no
possibility of such confusion exists and in areas of other muscles where
there is no possibility of extraneous electric pickup.

The abundance of data in Breinin's cases and in those of Walsh[139]
fully supports this concept.

The question arises whether stretch effects play a role in the discharge of the muscle in aberrant third nerve regeneration. It is improbable since the globe remains fixed; hence, stretch could not occur, nor could this explain the miosis or lid retraction.

The reinnervation potentials encountered may be due to the fact that a regenerating nerve fiber may innervate many more muscle fibers than is normally the case, producing a larger potential of longer duration.

DYSTHYROID OPHTHALMOPLEGIA (SEE FIGURE 31). The palsies associated with thyroid exophthalmos have been considered myopathies

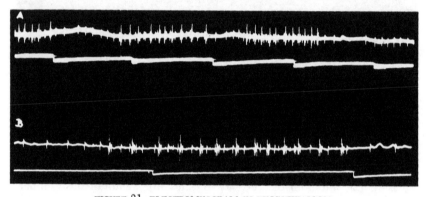

FIGURE 31. ELECTROMYOGRAM IN EXOPHTHALMOS

Upper trace, right superior rectus; *lower trace*, integrator. A, polyphasic and single units; B, polyphasic and single units at faster speed.

because of the appearance of characteristic pathologic changes in the muscle tissue. The electromyogram of the paretic extraocular muscles in early cases of non-congestive dysthyroid ophthalmoplegia reveals a normal innervational pattern. It is likely that the turgescence of the orbital tissues imposes some mechanical impediment to motility. With more advanced cases paretic patterns of innervation are seen, marked by poorly sustained irregular recruitment, polyphasic potentials, and good amplitude of units.[34]

It is possible that inflammatory or toxic effects upon the terminal axons are responsible for the palsies in the mild and moderately severe cases. Some authors consider a normal electric pattern in the presence of clinical palsy as evidence of myopathy.[111–114]

Exophthalmos alone does not produce muscle palsies or innervational disturbances. In the more severe congestive forms a shift in the electromyographic pattern to the myopathic type occurs. It is in such cases that the histologic changes of myopathy are encountered in the extraocular muscles. More refined methods of frequency analysis may reveal earlier myopathic changes than has hitherto been possible.[41]

Electromyographic and histologic studies of peripheral skeletal muscle involvement in advanced thyrotoxicosis show a well-marked myopathic pattern. It is of interest that the frequent involvement of the inferior rectus with adhesion to the floor of the orbit may present a pseudoparalysis relieved by surgery to that muscle.

LID RETRACTION. Lid retraction is an early characteristic finding in hyperthyroidism which has been investigated in a number of patients.[34,103] The inhibition of activity which normally occurs in downward gaze is no different in the retracted lid than in the normal muscle. Despite the complete absence of activity in the levator in gaze down, the lid maintains its retraction, which thus cannot be upon an innervational basis. Retrobulbar anesthesia and stellate ganglion block do not remove the retraction of the lid; therefore, it cannot be ascribed to either levator or sympathetic overaction. It is probable that intrinsic changes in the levator muscle are responsible for the retraction.[103]

MOEBIUS SYNDROME. Bilateral sixth and seventh nerve palsies constituting the Moebius syndrome have been attributed to aplasia of the nuclei. Multiple congenital defects are present, particularly the absence of limbs. A one-and-one-half-year-old infant was studied electromyographically.[34] Convergence was intact but there was only slight abduction. No horizontal version movements were elicited although vertical movements were good. The child substituted convergence for the version movement. The face was expressionless and there was no protective lid reflex to a threatening gesture. Electromyography of the lateral rectus revealed almost no potentials. Those that were seen were of extremely low amplitude and frequency. The orbicularis oculi and orbicularis oris revealed almost complete electric silence with only a few insertion potentials obtained from the latter. There was a suggestion of fibrosis during the insertion in the lateral rectus. The electromyographic pattern, multiple nerve involvement, and evidence of gaze palsy indicated a neurogenic lesion. The general picture was therefore suggestive of a congenital nuclear aplasia with supranuclear involvement.

Another report[138] on electromyography in the Moebius syndrome described insertion potentials, spindle pattern of innervation, and loss of reciprocity in the extraocular muscles, from which it was concluded that a supranuclear lesion was responsible. Biopsy of the lateral rectus was normal.

DUANE'S RETRACTION SYNDROME (SEE FIGURE 32). The etiology of the retraction syndrome has been variously ascribed to either the lateral or the medial rectus muscles. It is clear that the clinical entity can be

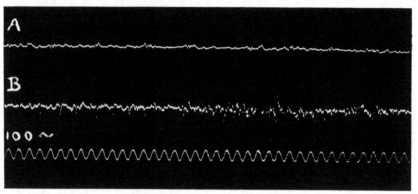

FIGURE 32. DUANE'S SYNDROME

A, lateral rectus, low-grade activity in primary position and attempted abduction; B, levator activity increases on attempted abduction.

produced by either fibrosis of the lateral rectus muscle or by anomalies associated with the medial rectus muscle. Electromyography permits an exact diagnosis of the disturbance to be made.[29] The lateral rectus has always shown an abnormal pattern varying from complete electric silence to a very low level of electric activity. The diagnosis has been confirmed by subsequent surgery in one case in which the lateral rectus was seen to be fibrotic and inelastic. In this patient the insertion of the electrode was attended by a gritty feeling clearly different from insertion into normal muscle. On several occasions such resistance has been experienced and the diagnosis could be made solely by the maneuver of electrode insertion. The medial rectus, levator, and inferior oblique muscles have fired normally in patients examined by Breinin.

In other studies,[7] both medial and lateral recti and even vertical muscles have been reported as abnormal. The figures presented are not convincing because of what appears to be inadequate technique. Furthermore, some of the patients described do not fit the concept of the Duane retraction syndrome. It is, nevertheless, entirely possible that some cases will exhibit innervational alterations of the internal rectus, but these are probably a minority.

Electromyography is of great value in determining the affected muscles in the Duane retraction syndrome. This is equally true of other fibrosis syndromes.

MYASTHENIA GRAVIS (SEE FIGURE 33). One of the most important applications of ocular electromyography is in the diagnosis of myasthenia gravis.[28,34,75] Because of the characteristic early involvement

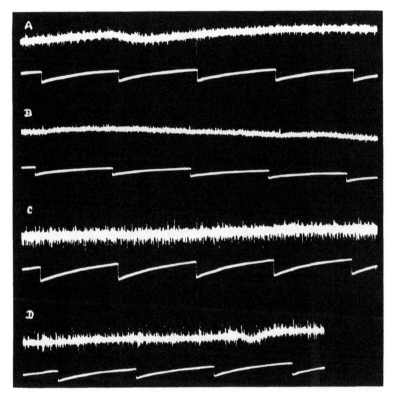

FIGURE 33. ELECTROMYOGRAM OF RIGHT LATERAL RECTUS IN MYASTHENIA GRAVIS

A, initial level; B, on protracted gaze right; C, 15 sec. after edrophonium was administered; D, 2 min. after edrophonium was administered.

of the extraocular muscles with varying degrees of ptosis and diplopia, these patients often present themselves first to the ophthalmologist. In many, the application of the standard pharmacologic tests such as prostigmine or intravenous edrophonium chloride (Tensilon®) will result in a prompt improvement in the clinical paresis. The diagnosis can thus be established on clinical grounds supported by pharmacologic testing. There are numerous cases, however, in which the pharmacologic tests are inconclusive. Ocular electromyography can, in many of these, establish the correct diagnosis.

The pattern of myasthenia gravis in the extraocular muscles is of a progressive decrease in activity of the muscle during sustained effort to maintain the gaze upon a given fixation point in the field of action of the muscle. It is expressed by a progressive fallout of motor units, such that the amplitude of the trace becomes progressively smaller until eventually it is virtually extinguished. This change does not appear to be produced by a decrease in size of the individual units but by a loss of those of higher amplitude until only small-amplitude units or none at all remain. This probably reflects the small innervation ratio and anatomical-pharmacologic uniformity of the motor units.

The fatigue pattern described above does not occur in other forms of extraocular muscle disease. In neurogenic palsies one may see a type of fatigue accompanied by irregular recruitment and paretic nystagmus bursts, but not the progressive fallout of activity so characteristic of myasthenia. In many patients this pattern alone is diagnostic. In advanced cases, the activity in the extraocular muscles is of a very low order, becoming almost extinguished.

The electromyographic pharmacologic test with edrophonium is by far the most delicate diagnostic tool available today. Breinin[28] employs the technique described by Osserman and Teng: 0.2 c.c. containing 2 mg. of the drug are administered intravenously over 15 sec. If there is no ocular response or cholinergic reaction, 0.8 c.c. more are then administered in 30 sec. This graded instillation of the drug limits the occurrence of cholinergic reactions (sweating, nausea, vomiting, abdominal pains, and collapse) as well as the occasional reaction of induced muscle weakness (false negative).

Responsive cases of myasthenia will exhibit a prompt reinnervation of the paretic muscles within 15 to 20 sec., which builds up to a maximum within a minute and then declines over two or three minutes more, sometimes even within the first minute, to the level existing prior to the administration of the drug. The importance of this electric response to edrophonium lies in the fact that the reaction appears pathognomonic of myasthenia and may occur in the complete absence of ocular movement. This means that the test can reveal cases which would be completely missed clinically. Not all patients exhibit a resurgence of activity, and in advanced cases degenerative changes in the muscles may preclude any pharmacologic response. As a rule, the most involved muscles should be tested. Occasionally a clinically normal muscle will reveal an abnormal pattern.

It is of interest that studies by Breinin[41] as well as Huber[74,75] have shown a myopathic pattern in some cases of myasthenia. The units are of low amplitude as a rule but may be large. This pattern will be described more fully under the section on progressive external ophthalmoplegia, but it clearly indicates a close association between the two entities. The failure of ocular movement in response to the drug despite an electric recovery also supports the notion of a myopathic process in the extraocular muscles in myasthenia gravis. Against this, however, is the observation that the mean duration of myasthenic units is often longer than normal units.[41]

Only two instances of mildly positive response to edrophonium in non-myasthenic cases have been encountered in patients exhibiting a dystrophic ophthalmoplegia. These may be dystrophic forms of myasthenia or myasthenic forms of dystrophy. The drug in one instance produced fasciculations and fibrillations in paretic extraocular muscle.[28]

Pulse height analysis[41] of myasthenic response to edrophonium shows a recovery of low-amplitude units first with progressive recovery of higher-amplitude units, the largest recovering last. These are the first to be lost as the drug wears off, and the electric pattern diminishes in reverse until only low amplitude or no activity remains.

Myasthenic patients to whom placebos were administered evidenced no alteration in electric activity. Some cases suspected of being myasthenia have been shown not to be so, because of typical non-myasthenic electric discharge patterns in extraocular muscle with and without pharmacologic testing.

OCULAR MYOPATHY (Progressive external ophthalmoplegia—primary muscular dystrophy). For many years the etiology of progressive external ophthalmoplegia was ascribed to lesions of the nuclei of the extraocular muscles. The extraordinary immobility of the eyes and ptosis associated with absent diplopia, commencing in early life and slowly progressing, evidences a genetic, abiotic defect. It is frequently observed in many members of a family, and such multiple involvements within families have been studied electromyographically.[34,41] Although the entity may be restricted to the extraocular muscles, it is not infrequently associated with peripheral dystrophic muscular changes and other congenital disturbances.[111,112] Tapetoretinal degeneration has also been associated with this entity.[41,136]

The electromyogram of the extraocular muscles in an advanced case typifies the myopathic process.[29,34,99,111] Myopathy, in contrast to neuropathy in which there is a loss of whole motor units, is characterized by a loss of the individual muscle fibers comprising the unit. Since these are the batteries of the unit, an action potential of diminished amplitude and shortened duration results. Increased numbers of polyphasic waves also occur. Despite the loss of the individual muscle fibers, the retention of the motor unit permits an intense interference pattern to be developed upon effort, and it is this combination of findings which characterizes intrinsic disease of the muscle. The electric pattern then is of a low amplitude and high frequency, with interference activity upon effort. This has a characteristic audio component, highpitched and rushing in sound, unlike any other form of ocular muscle disturbance. Despite the interference pattern, very little movement is produced on effort. Inveterate cases exhibit an extinction or near extinction of all electric activity in the extraocular muscles based upon the destruction of large numbers of muscle fibers.

Of great diagnostic interest is the fact that, in some individuals exhibiting severe loss of motility, the electric pattern appears quite normal with good or even increased amplitude and an abundance of potentials in the electromyogram.[111–112]

In 1955, Kamouchi[78] described myopathic potentials in extraocular muscle. Papst, Esslen, and Mertens[66,104–105,111–114] demonstrated the myopathic nature of progressive external ophthalmoplegia and inflammatory myopathy. In progressive external ophthalmoplegia they found an abundant discharge of normal-amplitude potentials in the extraocular muscles which contrasted with the almost complete ocular palsy of the patient. A careful examination of other muscles of the body showed the presence of a muscle dystrophy confirmed by histologic findings. The patient with inflammatory myositis also showed an abundance of potentials of normal amplitude. They concluded that the electromyographic diagnosis of myopathy consisted in finding an interference pattern of normal potentials in the presence of almost complete clinical paralysis whose degree was incompatible with such an electric picture, and in which there were no evidences of fibrillation or fasciculation.

A new form of ocular myositis was described[113] in which there may be little or no evidence of external inflammation of the eye, and in which paralysis of the extraocular muscles was correlated with a myopathic innervation pattern. They also pointed out the existence of a more acute inflammatory myositis with a similar electric pattern.

The quiet form of chronic ocular myositis was termed oligosymptomatic;[114] the acute form associated with pain, conjunctival inflammation, chemosis, and photophobia, resembling an exophthalmic ophthalmoplegia, was termed exophthalmic ocular myositis.[113] The former appeared related to the rheumatic collagen diseases (polymyositis).

Both conditions tended to spontaneous remissions and exacerbations and responded extraordinarily well to corticosteroid therapy.

In myositis, lid retraction so typical of endocrine exophthalmos was always absent and there were no other evidences of metabolic disturbance.

In endocrine exophthalmos, they detected only non-specific electromyographic alterations in extraocular muscle. The exophthalmic form of chronic ocular myositis must be distinguished from orbital tumor and endocrine exophthalmos by roentgenography and metabolic studies. They believe some cases of inflammatory pseudotumor of the orbit are really examples of exophthalmic myositis.

The authors reported amplitudes in the electromyogram up to 1 mv. with durations of about 1 msec. or less, although preponderantly amplitudes less than 100 μv. were recorded. It is extremely difficult to characterize these motor units as abnormal, since durations of 1 to 1.5 msec. occur commonly in normal extraocular muscle. A statistical increase of frequency and depression of amplitude would strengthen the diagnosis. To say that a normal electromyogram in the presence of a total clinical paralysis indicates myopathy does not provide a satisfactory criterion of the disease, although the surprising finding of apparently normal electric responses of myopathic muscle definitely occurs.

It must be concluded, therefore, that in the earlier phases of this disease the electromyogram is not diagnostic except by the process of exclusion, as they also noted. It is astonishing that such good electric activity can exist with such extreme loss of function. With the passing of time, the involvement of the muscle fibers proceeds to the stage wherein amplitudes are lowered and frequencies altered. Eventually, muscle degeneration results in the total loss of electric activity.

In an effort to resolve this problem, more refined spectrum (frequency) analysis techniques are being employed by Breinin.[41] Preliminary observations indicate a higher-frequency distribution in myopathy as compared with the normal or neuropathy. The myopathic frequency distribution, however, may also not be apparent in the earlier cases.

High-frequency shifts have been noted in the peripheral skeletal musculature in muscular dystrophy.[140] In peripheral muscles the dominant frequency in the normal and in neuropathy (100 to 250 cycles tailing off to zero at 800 cycles) was considerably lower than in myopathy, where a shift of the dominant frequency occurred to values above 400 cycles with an attenuation of low-frequency components. In normal facial and small hand muscles, a "broad spectrum" response occurred with a dominant frequency at 200 to 250 cycles and components extending up to 1500 cycles. This response was attributed to the high percentage of polyphasic potentials in those muscles.

SUPRANUCLEAR MECHANISMS (SEE FIGURES 34 AND 35). The primary role of electromyography is in the recognition of lower motor neurone disturbances. It records electric activity in the final common path. In

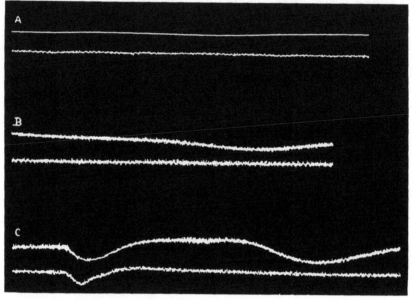

FIGURE 34. ELECTROMYOGRAM IN INTERNUCLEAR PALSY

Upper trace, right lateral rectus; *lower trace*, left medial rectus. A, gaze left, lateral rectus fully inhibited, medial rectus only partially; B, primary position; C, gaze right, spindle bursts in lateral rectus; constant level in medial rectus, same as in primary position.

peripheral skeletal muscle, supranuclear lesions are manifested chiefly by disturbances in the pattern of innervation rather than in the type of electric activity recorded. Thus, there are disturbances in reciprocity represented by cocontraction and synchrony of firing. The electromyographic study of the extraocular muscles in supranuclear lesions of man has demonstrated a number of frequently occurring findings.[36] These involve patterns of activity and not the character of the motor units involved. It should be clearly noted that the presence of these patterns is not *ipso facto* proof of supranuclear origin of the disturbance. The findings are merely suggestive and, in combination with

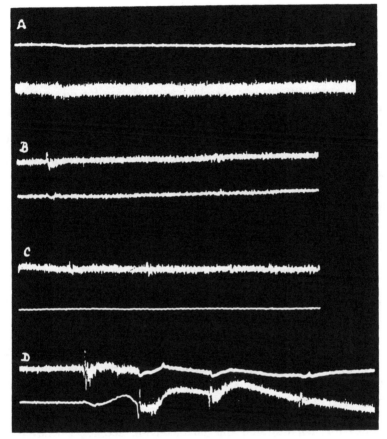

FIGURE 35. ELECTROMYOGRAM IN CONJUGATE DEVIATION

Upper trace, right medial rectus; *lower trace*, right lateral rectus. A, conjugate deviation, right; B, primary position; C, conjugate deviation, left, eyes closed; D, closed eyes to open eyes—conjugate deviation shifts from left to right.

clinical and other diagnostic modalities, permit another insight into the nature of the lesion. Furthermore, it is possible to have such patterns in other than supranuclear disturbances. Again, the electromyographic findings must be taken in the context of all the manifestations of the disease in the patient.

A frequent finding in supranuclear disturbances of extraocular muscle is a spindle pattern of innervation in which the discharge builds up to a peak and then declines in rhythmic fashion. This resembles the pattern of the electroencephalogram during sleep and barbiturate hypnosis. Such innervation spindles have also been observed in the extraocular muscles during sleep,[33] but have been encountered most frequently in gaze palsies or deviations. Pendular nystagmus exemplifies this pattern of spindle innervation. Another frequent finding in supranuclear disturbances is a saccadic pattern of innervation during versions. Such patterns may also be present during forced gaze movements and gaze disturbances. In conjugate deviations, saccadic patterns of innervation may occur in the horizontal recti.

Electromyographic study of the horizontal recti muscles in a patient with a cerebrovascular accident was instructive. With eyes open, there was conjugate deviation to the right. With the closing of the eyes, there was an immediate conjugate deviation to the left which had escaped the notice of the neurologists. The pattern was immediately obvious in the electromyogram and on inspection it appeared to be an example of the condition termed spastic deviation by Cogan.[47]

The presence of the electric findings of saccadic movement and spindle pattern may assist the ophthalmologist in establishing a diagnosis; thus, a supranuclear electric pattern of the antagonist in association with a lower motor neuron palsy of the agonist helped reveal the existence of a conjugate deviation that had escaped notice as a result of the masking effect of the peripheral palsy.

A patient with a brain tumor exhibited vertical oscillopsia. The electromyogram of the superior rectus revealed rhythmic spindle-type innervation patterns characteristic of gaze disturbances. This pattern was present in all levels of vertical gaze. A similar spindle pattern was encountered in a case of the jaw winking syndrome of Marcus Gunn. The levator demonstrated this characteristic activity whenever the tongue was touched to a particular part of the palate or when movements of the lower jaw to the opposite side were made. The strongest volitional discharge in the levator was much less than that which occurred during jaw or tongue movement.

Oculogyral crises in Parkinsonism are striking phenomena. Electromyography of the horizontal recti and vertical elevators demonstrated cocontraction as the eye rotated upward. It has been pointed out that cocontraction of the horizontal recti has been noted during retractory and convergence nystagmus.[29] That the cocontraction could be an artifact resulting from lid activity or movement has already been discussed. It should be pointed out that in the oculogyral crises the movement of the eye upwards is slow, and it is unlikely that electric activity from the lid could have played any significant part in this simultaneous activity.

Divergence Paralysis.—The question of the existence of a divergence center continues to exercise ophthalmologists and neurologists. A patient suspected of having a brain tumor developed a comitant esotropia greater for distance than near. No weakness of the lateral recti was noted at first. At the time of electromyographic examination, a definite paretic involvement of the left lateral rectus was present with some limitation of abduction. In view of this, the following findings must be taken with due reservation: "With the left eye fixing at near, the activity in the right lateral rectus was greater than it was when the left eye was fixing at distance." This innervational difference could, of course, be simply interpreted as reflecting the lesser angle of esotropia at near.

Internuclear Palsy.—The syndrome of the medial longitudinal fasciculus is frequently encountered in neuro-ophthalmologic practice and is generally attributable to multiple sclerosis or vascular lesions. Characteristically, the patient exhibits a failure of adduction of one or both medial recti with the retention of convergence in many cases. There is usually nystagmus of the abducted eye. Failure of adduction of the medial rectus is ascribed to supranuclear paralysis. No good explanation has been advanced for the characteristic nystagmus of the abducted eye. Electromyography has been extremely revealing in this syndrome. The failure of adduction is not a consequence of paresis of the medial rectus in the ordinary sense. The medial rectus exhibits recruitment up to a certain level and then abruptly ceases to increase its discharge despite attempted gaze into its field of action. There are absolutely no signs of paresis such as are encountered in lower motor disease and there is no detectable nystagmus of any degree.

The abduction nystagmus is a complex entity. In most cases the lateral rectus exhibits a spindle-type innervation with a pendular type of nystagmus. Jerky nystagmus may, however, occur with a paretic pattern of innervation. The former type probably represents supranuclear involvement; the latter nuclear involvement. Interruption of the supranuclear fiber to the contralateral medial rectus completely isolates this muscle from nystagmus innervation as well as gaze movement into its field of action. Where convergence is preserved, the medial rectus exhibits the normal convergence pattern of augmentation of activity from the primary position. In gaze out of the field of action of the apparently paretic medial rectus, reciprocal inhibition occurs in the usual fashion; on return of the gaze toward its field of action, it recruits up to the level of the primary position and then ceases to add an iota of innervation more, maintaining a constant tonic level which characterizes the muscle in the primary position. The antagonist lateral rectus is reciprocally inhibited as the eye rotates back toward the mid-line from the abducted position and may become completely inhibited in the primary position, in spite of which the eye fails to turn into the field of action of the firing medial rectus.

The syndrome of the medial longitudinal fasciculus reveals the existence of a *peripheral tonicity mechanism* isolated from supranuclear sources. The tonic firing of the medial rectus is not altered by the retention or absence of convergence ability.

It has already been pointed out that in normal saccadic movement, the rotation of the globe is dependent upon the activity of the agonist and ceases when the burst of the saccade is completed. The inhibition of the antagonist permits the movement to go on, but the antagonist plays no part in stopping the rotation. The abrupt cessation of movement under these conditions, with due allowance for minor overshoots and oscillations, reflects a natural resistance to rotation of the globe residing in mechanical factors of the orbit (muscular, elastic, fascial).[36,142]

In order to produce rotation of the globe, a steadily increasing amount of innervation is required in the agonist in order to overcome resistance to movement. The factor of such orbital resistance to rotation of the globe has not been adequately appreciated. In the syndrome described, the failure of the globe to rotate into the field of the medial rectus is attributable to the absence of augmentation of its agonist and not to faulty inhibition of its antagonist.

MECHANISM OF PARETIC STRABISMUS. The following theoretic relationship may be postulated. The extraocular muscles are associated in a system of homolateral and contralateral reciprocal innervation and reciprocal inhibition. Paretic strabismus is not a consequence of the loss of balanced pull between agonist and antagonist *per se*, although some mechanical, elastic balance does exist. Rather, it is the result of a disturbance of dynamic balance wherein loss of activity in the paretic muscle is associated with increased activity of the antagonist. This dynamic balance must be based on the integrity of lower motor centers and reflex arcs. It follows from this concept that paretic strabismus occurs only when the antagonist to the paretic muscle undergoes an increase in its level of innervation. In the absence of such an increased innervation the eye stands in the primary position. To be sure, an incomitant deviation will develop on gaze into the field of action of the paretic muscle, but on gaze away from the field of action of the paretic muscle there may be normal muscle balance. With the development of an imbalance in the adjustment, the antagonist to the paretic muscle undergoes an increase in its innervation, thus producing an angle of squint evident in the primary position and field of action of the antagonist as well. Undoubtedly, mechanical musculofascial factors exert some influence upon the balance, but this does not appear to be very great, and the angle of squint cannot be attributed in any great measure to such mechanical imbalance except for the subsequent development of contracture.

It is of interest that after procaine paralysis of a horizontal rectus the globe does not rotate into the field of the antagonist, nor is the innervation of the antagonist altered in the primary position. Such paralysis is not comparable with neurogenic palsies. There is probably a time factor involved in the alteration of innervation of paretic muscles.

In addition to the innervational features of paretic strabismus, the factor of contracture of the antagonist must be appreciated. The development of such a contracture alters the innervational picture and the character of the deviation, and it is perhaps for this reason that innervation changes of the antagonist in paretic strabismus have not been noted.[18]

It is probable that persistent overaction or contracture of the antagonist to a paretic muscle is more prejudicial to the eventual restoration of function than the paresis itself. Although the paresis may be removed completely in time, the contracture may persist indefinitely.

Innervational inhibition of the antagonist to a paretic muscle, however, does not seem impaired[17] and in the early phases of palsy may permit the globe to rotate back to the mid-line. With the development of contracture, although inhibition may still occur, the globe either remains in its deviated position or undergoes a lesser counter-rotation.

It should be further noted that supranuclear mechanisms are fully capable of altering the tonic activity of muscles and can cause the activity to fall to zero in the primary position.

COMITANT STRABISMUS. The study of comitant strabismus of childhood by electromyography is manifestly difficult because of the inapplicability of this technique to many children. Nevertheless, it is true that with patience one may secure excellent cooperation with reliable electromyographic testing. The phlegmatic child is a more satisfactory subject, whereas the hyperkinetic child will rarely permit the procedure. A useful gambit is to intrigue the child with the idea of "hearing the muscle speak." The electrode should not be brandished before his eyes but kept concealed.

The small amount of evidence available[18] indicates that the electric patterns of the horizontal recti in comitant strabismus resemble the normal, the difference being the deviated position of the eye. Rotations demonstrate normal patterns of reciprocity of agonists and antagonists. It does not seem probable that electromyography will cast much light upon the mechanisms of comitant strabismus.

An important exception to the above was the evidence supporting an active divergence mechanism derived from electromyographic investigation of intermittent exotropia.[26] It was unequivocally demonstrated that on breaking into exotropia the lateral rectus activity was augmented while the medial rectus activity was inhibited in the diverging eye. In connection with the physiologic investigations of vergence and other data, these findings helped to establish the basic law of innervation.

A/V SYNDROMES (SEE FIGURES 36 TO 39). Vertically incomitant horizontal squint has in the last few years become a topic of great interest.[137] A significant proportion of strabismus (15 to 25 percent

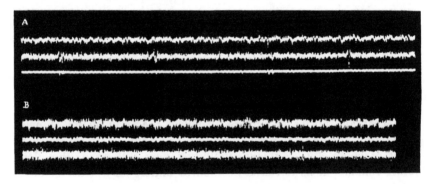

FIGURE 36. SIMULTANEOUS ELECTROMYOGRAPHY
Lateral rectus (*upper tracing*), medial rectus (*middle tracing*), and inferior oblique (*lower tracing*) in V exotropia. A, gaze down; B, gaze up.

according to Costenbader) exhibits such deviations. Several schools of thought have evolved, attributing the disturbance to over- or underaction of either the horizontal or the vertical muscles. According to the latter school, a V-type exotropia is considered to result from over-action of the inferior obliques which through their abducting component in elevation cause a horizontal divergence of the eyes which increases in upward gaze. On the basis of such concepts, surgery has been primarily addressed to the vertical muscles or in combination to vertical and horizontal muscles.

Breinin[34] pointed out that an electromyographic study in the A/V

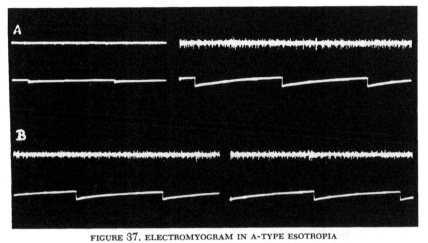

FIGURE 37. ELECTROMYOGRAM IN A-TYPE ESOTROPIA

Upper trace, right lateral rectus; *lower trace,* integrator. A, *left,* gaze up, slight activity; *right,* gaze down, good activity (O.S. fixing); B, *left,* O.D. straight up; *right,* O.D. straight down; no difference (O.D. fixing).

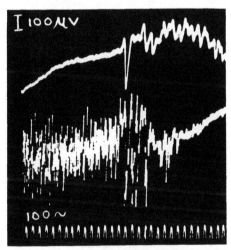

FIGURE 38. DIVERGENCE IN INTERMITTENT EXOTROPIA

Lateral rectus, *above;* medial rectus, *below.* On convergence the activity of the medial rectus increases, while the lateral rectus is increasingly inhibited. At the break there is marked activity in the lateral rectus which overlaps continued activity in the medial rectus for 20 msec. after which inhibition of the medial rectus occurs. The firing in the lateral rectus persists as long as the eye remains divergent.

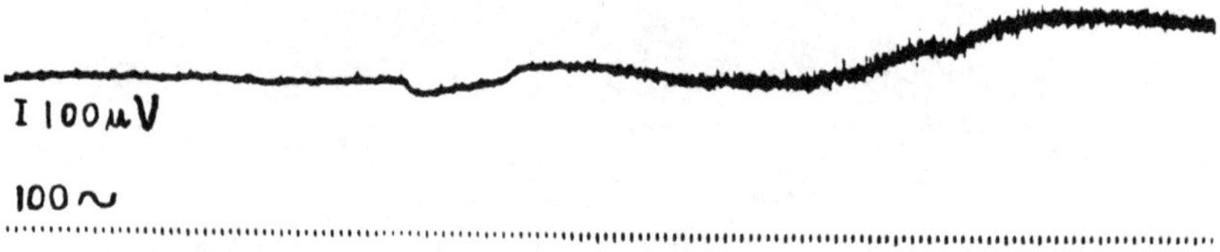

I 100μV

100 〜

FIGURE 39. INTERMITTENT EXOTROPIA WITH REMOTE FIXATION
Lateral rectus of diverging eye shows marked increase of firing as eye breaks from
fusion into exotropia.

syndromes showed an alteration in the innervation of the horizontal
recti which almost always accorded with the position of the eyes.
Thus, in V exotropia, the horizontal recti showed the reciprocal changes
characteristic of increasing divergence in upward gaze. Appropriate
changes were seen in the other categories of the A/V syndromes. At
the same time, the vertical movers showed the normal changes charac-
terizing muscles entering their field of activity.

These patients were studied with the deviating eye behind a cover,
so that fusion could not enter into the picture. As the fixing eye was
carried straight up, the deviating eye rotated upward and outward in
the V exotropia. The inferior oblique showed normal recruitment as the
eye entered into the upper field. As the eye rolled out, a marked
reciprocal change of innervation occurred in the horizontal recti with
the lateral rectus increasing and the medial rectus decreasing.

That the vertical muscles do not exhibit active innervational accessory abduction or adduction has been established, but that they have
such effects on a mechanical basis is undoubted.[31] These are entirely
consequences of the relation of the muscle plane to the center of
rotation. In gaze straight up or down through the primary position, the
horizontal recti show no significant change. Similarly, the vertical
recti show no change in rotations through the horizontal plane.
Although these findings have been generally confirmed,[109,130] some
variability in firing of the horizontal recti in vertical movements
through tertiary planes has been described.[132]

From the above observations, Breinin stated that the horizontal recti
must play some part in the varying angle of strabismus. In only a few
cases of the A/V syndromes originally examined did the horizontal
recti exhibit no particular change in vertical gaze. In these, the vertical
incomitancy was ascribed to the vertical muscles. From preliminary
observations it appeared wise to surgically attack the horizontal
muscles before the vertical ones, but where gross vertical imbalance
existed, classical rules should still be followed.

This statement is still sound advice, although it may have to be modified with increasing experience. The present conception of these entities is as follows. Both horizontal and vertical muscles play some part in the genesis of the A/V syndromes. The vertical muscles must exert a large mechanical effect which can be amplified through innervational alterations which increase the activity of such muscles in their fields of action. Such effects must be more pronounced in the torsional field of the vertical muscles where accessory duction effects are marked. In association with this mechanical effect of vertical muscles occurs an innervational change in the horizontal muscles of reciprocal nature which accords with the position taken by the eye. Whenever the eye rotates into a given position, there must be an appropriate alteration of innervation in all the muscles which normally carry the eye into that position. The concept of an innervational law of position has been presented and the alterations of the horizontal recti noted in the A/V syndromes may be explained as occurring in consonance with that innervational requirement.

It is impossible to say which of these sets of muscles has primacy in these actions. The syndromes may be altered by traditional vertical and horizontal muscle surgery, separately or combined. Vertical muscle surgery has a greater effect than horizontal surgery, but such surgery alone cannot remove the condition. Altering the placement of horizontal or vertical muscles on the globe alters the syndromes as well. Practically anything, it would appear, may effect a change in the A/V syndromes. No one factor appears solely responsible nor is any one procedure curative.

PHYSIOLOGY OF EXTRAOCULAR MUSCLE

The extraocular muscles have long been singled out as differing structurally and physiologically from other striated skeletal muscles of mammals. The nature of the muscle fiber, the presence of large amounts of elastic tissue and unusual nerve endings in the extraocular muscles, plus the marked pharmacologic sensitivity to acetylcholine, choline, and nicotine have been cited in placing the extraocular muscles in an intermediate position between the skeletal muscle of birds and amphibia and that of mammals.[42,61] Extraocular muscle is also said to demonstrate an affinity with smooth muscle.[42]

Furthermore, the anatomical and histologic distinctions of extraocular muscle, its low innervation ratio, variety of nerves and nerve endings, and membrane permeability[61] characteristics have been adduced in explanation of certain aspects of ocular motility. Differences in the characteristics of saccadic and vergence movements, for example, have been attributed to a dual (somatic and autonomic) innervation of extraocular muscle. In addition to large myelinated somatic efferent nerves, extraocular muscle possesses many small-diameter, non-myelinated fibers which are presumed to be visceral efferents. A unique tension-producing role has been proposed for the latter.[4] Both large and small muscle fibers are present in extraocular muscle.

We have been unable to demonstrate the functional existence of a hypothetical dual innervation or the presence in extraocular muscle of a slow muscle fiber contraction system.

The characteristically sustained tonic activity of extraocular muscle in the waking state has been related to interaction of muscle feedback and the reticular activation system of the brain stem.

The presence of muscle spindles and typical spindle discharge responses to stretch[50] and the existence of a gamma efferent system[144] in extraocular muscles indicate a fundamental kinship with peripheral skeletal muscle. The following findings of basic similarities in chemical response and contractile properties of the two types of muscle do not support the concept of extraocular muscle uniqueness.

All studies tend to show that differences between eye muscle and limb muscle are quantitative rather than qualitative and may be considered modifications related to the highly specialized nature of eye movement.

Acetylcholine *in vivo* and *in vitro* elicits a sharp contraction of extraocular muscle whereas choline and nicotine are said to produce a slower, more protracted contraction.[61] It is pointed out that the peripheral skeletal muscles of mammals do not exhibit these responses unless they are denervated or are embryonal prior to the time of their innervation. Acetylcholine elicits a tetanic contraction of extraocular muscle. Eserine produces similar effects on extraocular muscle as on peripheral musculature. A single nerve volley will produce a series of decrementing discharges. After eserinization, both acetylcholine and repetitive nerve stimulation evoke a contracture which blocks the propagation of excitation along the muscle fiber.[42] Acetylcholine elicits contracture in denervated extraocular muscle and this effect is also produced in normal extraocular muscle by succinylcholine and decamethonium.[7,73,91]

The extreme sensitivity of the extraocular muscles to curare is well known. This sensitivity is attributed to a much greater uniformity in threshold and sensitivity of the fibers of eye muscle than those of peripheral musculature. Hence, a small depression of excitability would exclude a very large number of fibers, or all, from response to a nerve volley.[42]

PHARMACOLOGIC STUDIES. A number of drug studies were made in animals (cat and dog) in order to assess the physiologic differences of eye muscles from other skeletal muscles.[40] From these experiments arose problems of (*a*) how the drug reaches the muscle, (*b*) saturation time of the drug on the muscle studied, and (*c*) the meaning of such drug studies in consideration of the physiology of the whole animal, for example, peripheral vs. central activation.

The importance of the over-all physiologic study has not received adequate emphasis. Central nervous system effects may overshadow peripheral effects. In many of the following studies, cardiorespiratory and electroencephalographic records were obtained as well as peripheral and extraocular myograms and electromyograms.

Epinephrine.—The possibility that small-diameter nerve fibers found in extraocular muscle constituted part of an autonomic motor mechanism to tension-producing elements was investigated. If these fibers were components of the sympathetic system, then they should respond to stimulation of the cervical sympathetic trunk with a rise in muscle tension. Further, one would expect increased tension with epinephrine injection. There is, however, a complete absence of effect on the inferior oblique during supramaximal cervical sympathetic stimulation (Figure 40, top).

Epinephrine also fails to elicit muscle contraction (Figure 41, center). Epinephrine in massive doses injected directly into the carotid artery produced no measurable change in the rest tension of the inferior oblique, lateral or medial rectus, while changes in the epinephrine-sensitive structures of the orbit (nictitating membrane, pupil) were readily observable. The observations on cervical sympathetic stimulation agree with results reported previously.[25,146]

If the small-diameter fibers in extraocular muscle were components of the parasympathetic system, differentiation from the somatic system would be difficult since, in both, the neuromuscular transmitter is acetylcholine.

Acetylcholine.—Topical application of *acetylcholine* produced no effect on extraocular muscle in either the cat or the dog. Administration intravenously, or intra-arterially via the lingual artery back into the carotid, produced variable effects depending on dosage from no measurable change to strong spontaneous activity lasting up to five minutes. In addition, with high dosage the face or scalp muscles were also affected as shown by visible movement, twitching of the vibrissae,

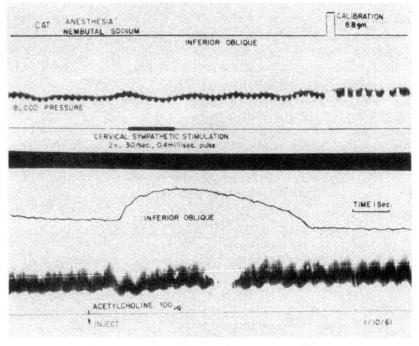

FIGURE 40

Top, absence of inferior oblique response to cervical sympathetic stimulation in the cat; *bottom*, effect of acetylcholine on tension. (*Artifact*: Bottom record, blood pressure trace, elevation due to previous injection.)

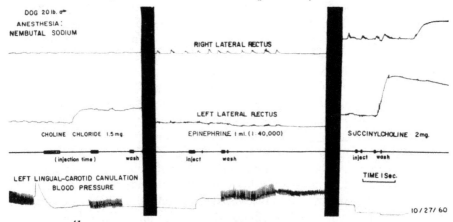

FIGURE 41. COMPARATIVE EFFECT OF CHOLINE, EPINEPHRINE, AND SUCCINYLCHOLINE ON EYE MUSCLE TENSION

(*Artifacts*: Small deflections in middle and last trace of eye muscle gauge due to strong respiration movement. Artifacts in blood pressure trace due to manipulation of common cannula for pressure registration and drug injection.)

and strong muscle interference with the electroencephalogram recording (Figures 42 to 44).

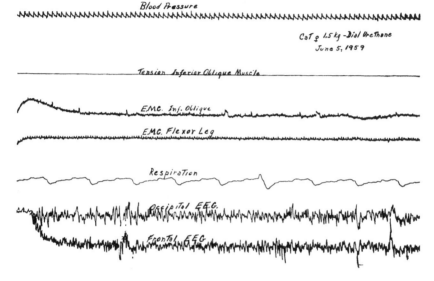

FIGURE 42. CAT CONTROL RECORD

Traces of direct blood pressure from left carotid cannula; strain gauge tension of eye muscle; EMG from bipolar recording electrodes of eye and leg muscles; thermistor (inside cannula) record of respiration from tracheal cannula; two EEG monopolar recordings.

The effect of blood supply on muscle innervation was often more significant than the effect of the drug. Prolonged carotid occlusion depressed the muscle activity and tension. Intravenous injection produced transient effects on eye muscle with larger dosage but this was overshadowed by the strong effects on the central nervous system. The EEG records were not affected in the moderately anesthetized cat or dog except at high dosage levels. Maximal electric activity and rise in tension of ocular muscle were observed at dosage levels which completely flattened the electroencephalogram. The EEG leads were both monopolar from frontal, parietal, and occipital areas as well as bipolar from homologous areas.

A more sensitive indication of acetylcholine effect was manifested by central nervous system activity as well as a general peripheral effect as shown by direct blood pressure and respiratory recordings. Intravenous injection produced only a slight transient effect in one animal but a serious depression of vital signs in six other animals.

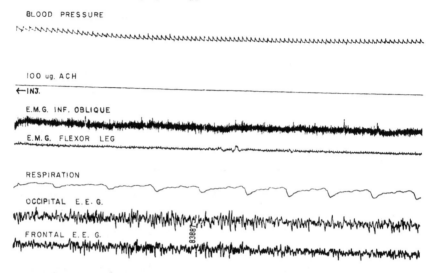

FIGURE 43. RECORDING AFTER LINGUAL CANNULATION INTO CAROTID ARTERY

Injection of 100 μg. acetylcholine. Note decrease in blood pressure, stimulatory action on eye muscle, and slow respiration. A rise in eye muscle tension occurred but the myogram channel was not recording. A slight increase in leg EMG occurred. No measurable effect on the EEG at this dosage level is seen.

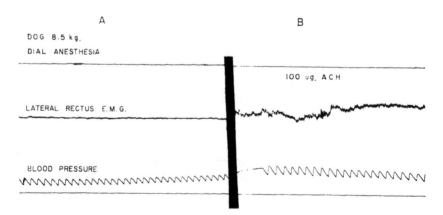

FIGURE 44. DOG

A, control record of lateral rectus EMG and blood pressure; B, effect of acetylcholine via carotid artery injection. Note strong stimulatory action on muscle, increase in blood pressure, and marked decrease in heart rate (initial flat line of blood pressure is artifact).

Attempts were made to determine the effect of acetylcholine on peripheral muscle in these experiments. Usually a flexor muscle of the forelimb was tested. By carotid injection, in only one experiment were a strong increase in the electromyogram and rise in tension observed and this only with a large overdose. More often a fibrillary twitching was observed by inspection of the animal. The most striking effects were on the muscles of the face and scalp, especially movement of the vibrissae which paralleled the eye muscle activity with lingual artery injection of acetylcholine. The transient stimulatory action on respiration was also a sensitive indicator.

Although these experiments appear to confirm previously held ideas that extraocular muscle is more sensitive to acetylcholine than are peripheral limb muscles, the experimental methods supporting this conclusion must be taken into consideration: An injection via the carotid of acetylcholine completely floods the eye muscle substance simultaneously. Only by close arterial injection can the whole of a peripheral skeletal muscle be flooded as quickly and efficiently as can an ocular muscle. The size of peripheral muscle is usually much greater and thus sampling of slight electric activity is less efficient. Also, effector sites are relatively fewer in peripheral muscle and spread over a larger mass.

Using close arterial injection a gross comparison was made of the acetylcholine effect in extraocular and limb muscle. An injection of 80 μg. of acetylcholine into the carotid regularly produced maximal contraction of extraocular muscles (Figure 45). The drug was administered with a hypodermic syringe through a polyethylene cannula tied into the stump of the lingual artery. The response is seen as a double contraction, the second hump occurring as the residuum in the cannula was washed in with saline. Using a modification of the technique of Rowley, Wells, and Irwin[147] for arterial injection of the anterior tibial muscle, 80 μg. of acetylcholine injected into the popliteal artery also produced a strong contraction of the anterior tibial muscle (Figure 46). With intracarotid injection, it usually required about 30–50 μg. of acetylcholine to produce a significant ocular muscle contraction, while as Rowley *et al.*[147] reported, anterior tibial contraction may be produced with as little as 2–5 μg. of acetylcholine (Figure 48). It is difficult to draw conclusions as to the relative sensitivity of ocular and limb muscle to acetylcholine since their responses are affected so largely by the techniques employed. It is clear, however, that both types of muscle respond briskly to minute amounts of acetylcholine.

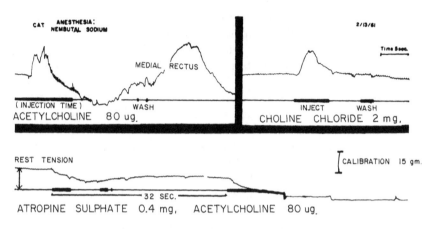

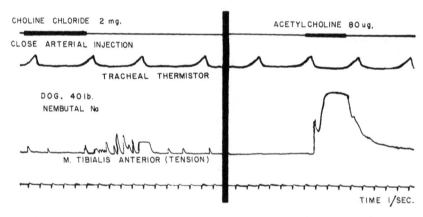

FIGURE 45

Top, comparative effect of acetylcholine and choline on eye muscle; *bottom,* short-term blocking action of atropine on acetylcholine injection.

FIGURE 46. COMPARATIVE EFFECT OF INTRA-ARTERIAL INJECTION OF CHOLINE AND ACETYLCHOLINE ON LIMB MUSCLE OF THE DOG

(*Artifact:* The flat top of the tension trace indicates overload of recording mechanism.)

Atropine.—Topical application of *atropine* produced no effect on extraocular muscle. A slight initial stimulating effect on the resting tonic activity followed by a short-term block was seen with bipolar recording in the intact preparation after intra-arterial administration. This could not be explained as an effect of the central nervous system

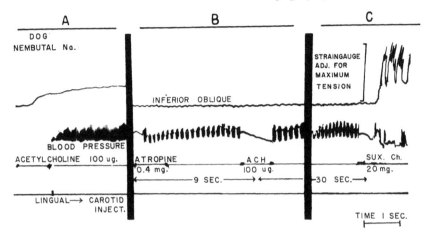

FIGURE 47. EFFECT OF ATROPINE AS A SHORT-TERM BLOCKING AGENT ON A SUB-
SEQUENT INJECTION OF ACETYLCHOLINE BUT NOT ON SUCCINYLCHOLINE; MEDIAL AND
LATERAL RECTUS MUSCLES IN THE CAT

A, control and effect of acetylcholine, tension present; B, atropine followed nine
seconds later by acetylcholine, no tension; C, atropine followed by succinylcholine,
tension produced.

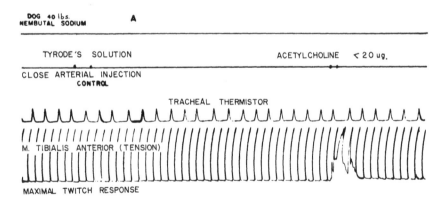

FIGURE 48. CONTROL FOR TESTING EFFECTS OF ATROPINE (SEE ALSO FIGURES 49 AND
50) ON ENDOGENOUS (TRANSMITTER AGENT) AND EXOGENOUS ACETYLCHOLINE

Endogenous acetylcholine release via nerve stimulation, exogenous acetylcholine
via injection in carotid artery. Tyrode's solution (control) shows no effect on
spontaneous tension or evoked tension. Small acetylcholine injection produces
spontaneous tension. Limb muscle, tibialis anterior, of the dog.

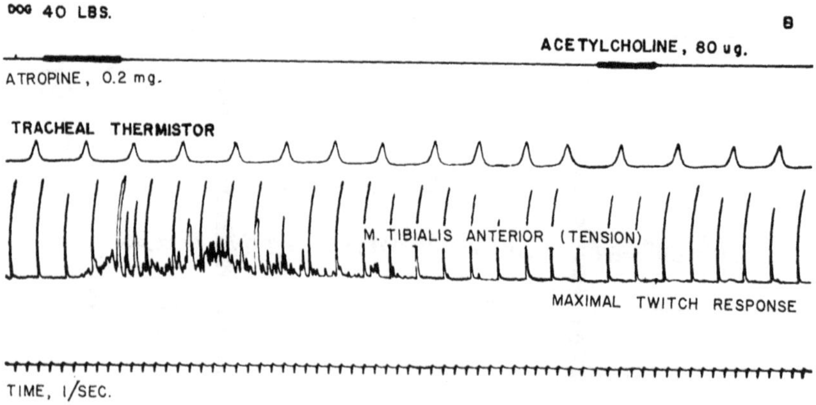

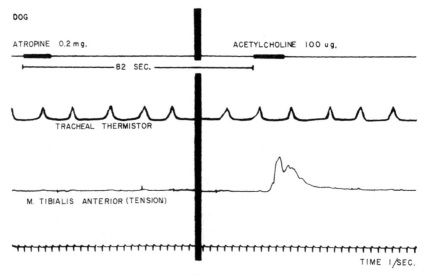

FIGURE 49. EFFECT OF ATROPINE AS A SHORT-TERM BLOCK ON EXOGENOUS BUT NOT
ENDOGENOUS ACETYLCHOLINE

Note also additional slight irritative effect of atropine. (Control, Figure 48.)

FIGURE 50. ILLUSTRATION OF SHORT-TERM EFFECT OF ATROPINE BLOCK

Above shows return of acetylcholine response after atropine block has partially
subsided. (See also Figures 48 and 49.)

acting on the eye muscle through the intact nerve supply since it
persisted after denervation. Subsequent acetylcholine injection had no
stimulating effect through the short-lived atropine block (Figures 45
and 47). Succinylcholine, however, overcame the block (Figure 47).

Similar responses occurred in anterior tibial muscle with close arterial injection. Although atropine blocked exogenous acetylcholine for over a minute, at no time did it prevent the action of endogenous acetylcholine (twitch contraction with nerve stimulation) (Figures 48 to 50).

Choline.—Choline, the hydrolytic product of acetylcholine, is said to produce a slow tonic contraction of extraocular muscle and to be without effect on innervated skeletal muscle.[61] Figure 45 shows the contractile effect on the medial rectus of injected choline chloride and acetylcholine. Although choline is relatively a poor stimulant since the amount required here is 50–100 times as great as for acetylcholine, the muscle response is brisk. A definite contractile effect of this amount of choline on the anterior tibial muscle (with close arterial injection) is clearly seen in Figure 46.

Nicotine.—Nicotine is also believed to exert different effects on extraocular and peripheral skeletal muscle.[61] It is stated that nicotine will stimulate intact extraocular muscle but not peripheral skeletal muscle, except following denervation sensitization.[1] Nicotine, by intravenous or intracarotid injection, stimulates extraocular muscle at dosage levels which do not affect peripheral skeletal muscle (Figure 51). Using the above-mentioned techniques, a powerful action on

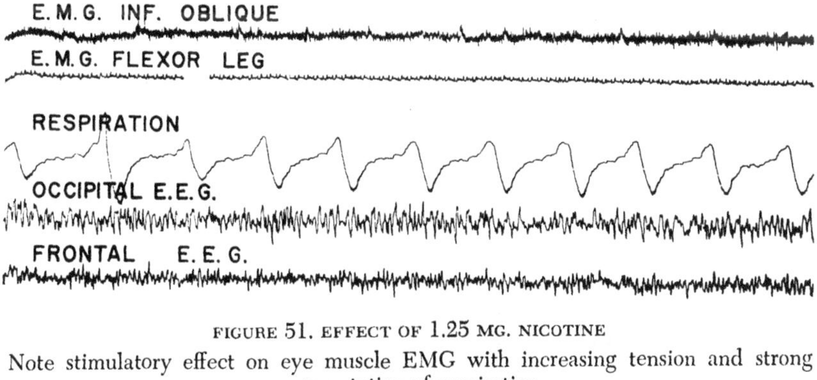

FIGURE 51. EFFECT OF 1.25 MG. NICOTINE

Note stimulatory effect on eye muscle EMG with increasing tension and strong augmentation of respiration.

extraocular muscle of an intracarotid injection of 1 cc. of nicotine in a 0.1 percent solution in saline is evident (Figure 52, top). With close arterial injection, however, one-half this amount can produce a strong contraction in the normal anterior tibial muscle (Figure 52, bottom).

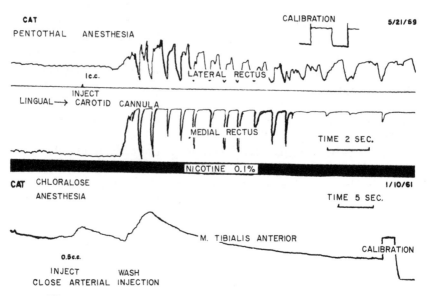

FIGURE 52. EFFECT OF NICOTINE INJECTION ON EYE AND LIMB MUSCLE IN THE CAT

Succinylcholine.—Succinylcholine is a depolarizing agent like acetylcholine, but, unlike the latter, it is not rapidly destroyed by true cholinesterase and therefore remains in the vicinity of the motor endplate until it diffuses into the blood stream where it is hydrolyzed in the presence of the serum pseudocholinesterase. Its action is prolonged by eserine.

Contraction of the extraocular muscles by succinylcholine and to a lesser degree by decamethonium had been noted by Hofmann and Lembeck[73] in 1952. In 1953, Hofmann and Holzer[72] reported that succinylcholine elevated the intraocular pressure. The globe was also noted to rotate into a divergent position and to remain fixed there. They suggested that the elevated intraocular tension was caused by a contraction of the extraocular muscles.

In 1955, Lincoff *et al.*[92] showed that the intraocular pressure was elevated by succinylcholine in man and in the cat. The effect was minimized or obliterated by deep general anesthesia. Isolated extraocular muscles in the cat were seen to be contracted by the drug. When all but one of the extraocular muscles were severed from the globe, the eye rotated into the field of action of the intact muscle following administration of the drug. It was concluded that the action of succinylcholine was to produce contraction of the extraocular muscles, thereby compressing the globe and elevating the intraocular pressure.

In 1957, Lincoff, Breinin, and De Voe[91] demonstrated the effect of succinylcholine on the extraocular muscles of cat, dog, and man. Succinylcholine in the dog and cat produced a state of contracture in the inferior oblique muscle with decreased twitches in response to stimulation. A more complete loss of response to twitch was demonstrated in the gastrocnemius, but no contracture was evident in that peripheral muscle.

Electromyography of cats under sodium pentothal anesthesia demonstrated that succinylcholine elicited bursts of high-frequency action potentials of low amplitude maintained for several minutes and then disappearing. The electromyogram in man showed an identical response of the extraocular muscle. High-frequency, low-amplitude potentials were elicited by the drug for several minutes following which electric silence ensued. Under deep levels of general anesthesia this effect was blocked, although fasciculations and flaccid paralysis of the peripheral skeletal musculature occurred. The onset of the effect on the intraocular pressure occurred within 10 to 20 sec., lasting for a total of about two to three minutes. The electromyographic response occurred in about 10 sec. and disappeared within one to two minutes. The firing response lasted for only 30 sec. in some instances. It was concluded that the use of succinylcholine was inadvisable in intraocular surgery because of compression of the globe. It was further concluded that the action of succinylcholine in elevating intraocular pressure was due to a sustained contracture induced in the extraocular muscle, but that this effect was minimized in deeply anesthetized patients.

In 1957, Dillon and associates[57] studied the action of succinylcholine on extraocular muscles and intraocular pressure. Strips of extraocular muscle of a cat and man demonstrated a contracture following the instillation of succinylcholine. Small doses of the drug at intervals produced a step-like contraction. In large doses, following an initial high tension, a complete block occurred. Decamethonium in the cat produced the same level of contracture as acetylcholine, but had a lesser effect in man. They also concluded that since intraocular pressure is raised by succinylcholine there was danger in its use in ocular surgery.

In 1957, Bjork and associates[20] observed enophthalmos elicited by succinylcholine and reported their observations on the use of succinylcholine and noradrenaline on the intraorbital muscles. They observed the development of enophthalmos in man and in the rat, produced about 20 sec. after instillation of the drug, lasting four to five minutes.

Electromyograms demonstrated a low-level activity elicited by succinylcholine lasting for some one-half to one minute, following which silence developed. They ruled out contraction of the extraocular muscles as a cause of the retraction of the globe because of the low-level electric activity. They concluded that there was a possibility of contracture but that it was not probable. They demonstrated an opposing action upon the nictitating membrane of noradrenaline and succinylcholine and concluded that the action of the latter was not upon the extraocular muscles but upon the smooth muscle of the orbit, which had not been taken into consideration before. The effect on the smooth musculature of the orbit, they concluded, was decisive in producing the retraction of the globe and other effects. They also reported that enophthalmos in man occurred in stage 3, plane 2, of general anesthesia with succinylcholine.

In an effort to resolve some of these conflicting viewpoints, a study was undertaken on the action of succinylcholine upon the extraocular muscles of the experimental animal[41] and in man,[40] using electromyography and strain gauge tension recording. The blocking effect of succinylcholine upon a nerve muscle preparation of the inferior oblique was readily demonstrated with a non-electric contracture developing in the muscle. It was apparent in these studies that the block was due to a sustained muscle depolarization, since there was no response to subsequent nerve stimulation or injection of acetylcholine in large doses. The effect began within 10 sec. and lasted from 2 to 15 minutes (Figures 53 to 58). Decamethonium and hexamethonium also produced contracture (Figure 59).

In order to study the tension produced by contracting extraocular muscle, a strain gauge was devised which could be employed in testing the extraocular muscles of man and animals. For use in man, the strain gauge (Statham) was mounted upon a headband taken from a Schepens binocular ophthalmoscope. In this way, movements of the subject's head did not produce artifactual response of the gauge. The procedure is done during surgery. The muscle to be tested is isolated from the globe and its tendon hooked up to the strain gauge with fine wire (Figure 60).

In the animal, instillation of the drug produced the usual depolarization bursts for a minute, which then disappeared leaving electric

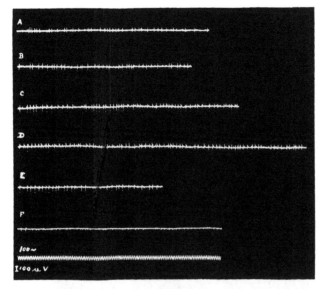

FIGURE 53. EFFECT OF SUCCINYLCHOLINE CHLORIDE IN MAN

A, before administration of drug; B, C, D, E, 15 sec. to 2 min.
later (increased frequency and amplitude); F, after 2 min.,
almost silent.

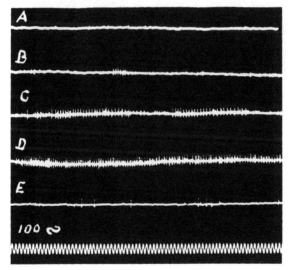

FIGURE 54. EFFECT OF SUCCINYLCHOLINE CHLORIDE IN THE
CAT

A, before administration of drug; B, C, D, 15 sec. to 1 min.
later (increased frequency and amplitude); E, after 1½ min.,
almost silent.

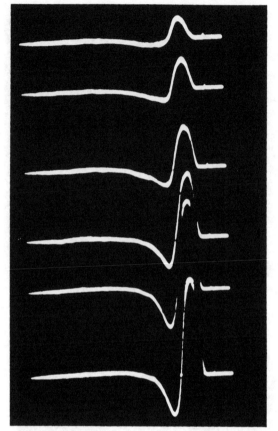

FIGURE 55. NERVE-MUSCLE PREPARATION OF INFERIOR
OBLIQUE
EMG shows development of neuromuscular block to
single shock nerve stimulation after succinylcholine.

silence. The strain gauge tension went up within seconds after instillation and remained at a very high level for several minutes; at times it
lasted 10 to 15 minutes. This demonstrated that true non-electric
contracture occurred.

With the strain gauge technique during general anesthesia, instillation of succinylcholine elicited a prompt contracture of high degree
in the extraocular muscle of man, lasting some two to three minutes
(Figures 61 and 62). Subsequent injections elicited a similar rise
of tension. These studies demonstrated that the action of the drug in
raising intraocular pressure was due to its effect upon the extraocular
muscles which underwent contracture thereby compressing the globe.

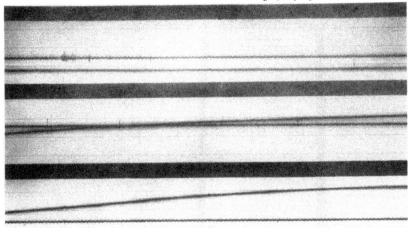

FIGURE 56. OSCILLOSCOPE RECORD OF CAT R.L.R. SHOWING STATE OF CONTRACTURE
FOLLOWING SUCCINYLCHOLINE

EMG, *upper trace*; myogram, *lower trace*. Brief burst in muscle followed by
electric silence and sustained contracture after succinylcholine.

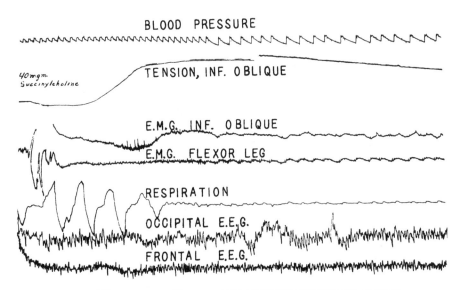

FIGURE 57. EFFECT OF 40 MG. SUCCINYLCHOLINE INJECTED VIA CAROTID

Note decrease in heart rate, arrest of respiration, large sustained rise in strain
gauge tension of eye muscle. A brief burst of activity in eye muscle is followed
by electric silence (contracture). Little change in EEG record.

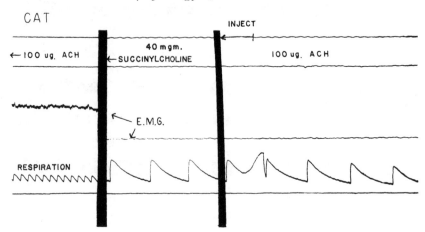

FIGURE 58. EFFECT OF ACETYLCHOLINE FOLLOWED BY 40 MG. SUCCINYLCHOLINE AND
A SUBSEQUENT INJECTION OF ACETYLCHOLINE
After succinylcholine block, acetylcholine had no effect.

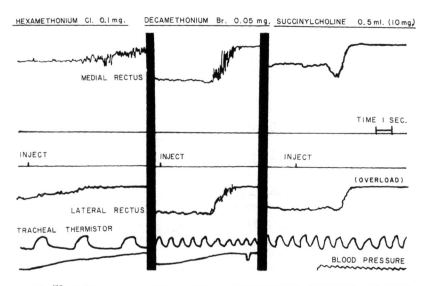

FIGURE 59. COMPARATIVE EFFECT OF AN INTRACAROTID INJECTION OF HEXA-
METHONIUM CHLORIDE, DECAMETHONIUM BROMIDE, AND SUCCINYLCHOLINE ON THE
PRODUCTION OF TENSION IN THE MEDIAL AND LATERAL RECTUS MUSCLE OF THE
EYE IN THE DOG.

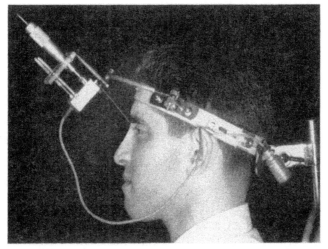

FIGURE 60. STRAIN GAUGE ASSEMBLY AND HEAD BAND IN HUMAN
OPERATIONS
Unit provides maximum rigidity; yet gauge may be placed in
plane of any eye muscle. Electrically isolated tungsten wire
connects gauge with muscle.

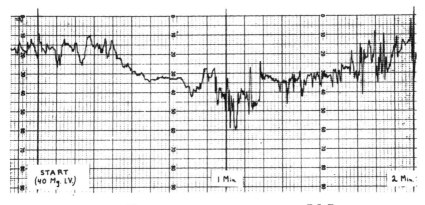

START
(40 Mg. I.V.)   1 Min.   2 Min.

FIGURE 61. HUMAN STRAIN GAUGE RECORD OF R.L.R.
Indicating that contracture from succinylcholine occurred within 30 sec. and
lasted over a period of 2 min.

It is clear that the mechanism suggested by Bjork and associates[20]
is untenable. Whatever effect there is upon smooth muscle of the
orbit can play little part in the observed action of succinylcholine upon
intraocular pressure; the very concept they rejected, namely, contracture, is the mechanism of action.

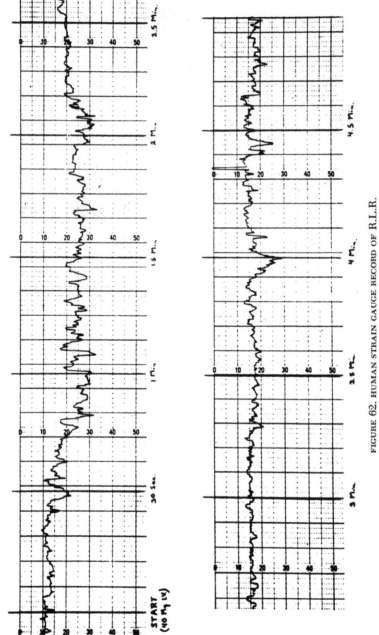

FIGURE 62. HUMAN STRAIN GAUGE RECORD OF R.L.R.

Indicating that maximum contracture effect from succinylcholine occurred after 1 min. and persisted over 5 min.

ELECTRODE-MUSCLE RELATIONS. A basic problem concerns the relation of electrode to the muscle as a method of sampling activity. Several important questions arise:

(*a*) As the concentric bipolar electrode records from a restricted field of activity, is it possible that this would produce data with a substantial error for assessing general muscle activity? This does not appear to be the case in peripheral muscle.[76]

(*b*) What are the advantages and disadvantages of small and large bipolar electrodes on the recorded information as opposed to mono-polar-type information?

(*c*) As the muscle shortens, is there a shift of electrode position sufficient that the field of sample may be altered?

Experiments performed to answer these questions were made on cat eye muscles supplemented by observations on the dog, both in the intact preparation and with the muscles detached and the globe enucleated.

Monopolar recording was made with one electrode in the belly of the muscle and the reference electrode at the killed end of the tendon insertion.

Bipolar records were made with two active electrodes placed with different interelectrode distances in the muscle mass.

Concentric electrode records were made with insulated and non-insulated barrels ranging from 20 to 31 gauge. Strain gauges were tied at the tendon insertion to check on the extent of mechanical con-traction as well as to indicate the onset of activity. Both the spon-taneous and evoked potentials were compared by these methods.

Monopolar recording results.—Although this method is successful in recording a greater amount of activity than any other method, the wide field sampling made it difficult to distinguish an increase of activity during muscle contraction from the spontaneous background firing. Also, because of greater tissue-electrode resistance and distance from electrode to individual muscle fibers, greater amplification was necessary, which increased random noise and electrode contact pop-ping. One of the most serious difficulties with electrodes distantly separated or contacting different tissue was electrode polarization. Attempts were made to decrease this by using Ag–AgCl electrodes; however, during muscle contraction with high amplification, muscle DC polarization potentials are often larger than the spiking electro-myogram potentials. Of course, the DC shift may be canceled by applying an opposing current in the resting preparation but not during the phasic DC shift of muscle contraction.

Concentric electrode results.—Although large, uninsulated concentric needles gave a slightly greater sampling, the interference pattern of excessive sampling itself tended to obscure the relative increase in the over-all electromyogram during contraction. Secondly, because of injury, probing for optimum sites for muscle-electrode positioning was limited. On the other hand, working with finer and finer insulated electrodes decreased the field pickup to the point where excessive probing was often necessary, and apart from single unit pickup it added little to the assessment of muscle activity. The data obtained with concentric electrodes correlated well with tension in extraocular muscle.

Point contact results.—Very fine needles insulated to the tip, of less than 0.5 cm. in total length, connected by the lightest "hair" wire were used as floating contacts on the surface or plunged into the muscle substance, in an attempt to minimize contact shift during muscle contraction. However, it was found that the varying relation of the contractile substance to its surrounding connective tissue produced, with this "negligible-mass" electrode, as much shift as with the larger standard variety. In addition, the decrease in size of the electrode contact increased muscle-electrode resistance. This required higher amplification with the attendant problem of amplifier noise and RF interference. The small "hair-wire" connection increased stray capacitance to ground, which tended to round off the spike potential and decrease its size owing to its high frequency. (Future work using a cathode follower probe will overcome part of this difficulty.)

Conclusions.—The ordinary 30- to 31-gauge, stainless steel, concentric needle electrode, large enough to have sufficient strength to penetrate dense connective tissue with relative ease, is small enough not to produce excessive injury and samples a sufficiently large field to produce a close correlation to strength of contraction. At the same time, it has a restricted enough field so that a slight increase in activity is less obscure by the formation of recorded envelopes and phasic cancellation. Electrode shift during eye movement is a minor problem in the intact preparation but becomes more of a problem when the muscle is detached from the globe and allowed to undergo excessive shortening. However, point contact shift changes the pattern sufficiently so that it is apparent to the experienced investigator.

The recording of spontaneous muscle activity with monopolar methods was found to be inefficient. As only a small percentage of fibers, not necessarily adjacent, within the muscle mass are in continuous activity in the animal, the increase in distance from foci of activity with the monopolar electrode required higher amplification with the attendant difficulties as stated above.

No evidence was found by these methods to uphold the old theory of "rotation of muscle activity" from one fiber to another due to a fatigue factor. A motor unit displaying a certain, continuous firing rate of spontaneous activity greatly increased its rate during phasic muscle contraction. Other units showing no resting activity would fire only during phasic muscle contraction and then returned to their previous state of silence.

Monopolar recording was found to be of value primarily with synchronous evoked activity through nerve stimulation. The effects of drug dilution producing fractional neuromuscular blocks were easier to determine by this method. When a drug produced a partial neuro-muscular block or affected part of the contractile mechanism, the height of the combined action potentials or total strength of contraction from nerve or direct muscle stimulation could be compared with the stable control level.

DYNAMICS OF CONTRACTION. One of the most striking peculiarities of eye muscle in comparison with limb skeletal muscle is the speed of contraction and relaxation.[42,51] In order to investigate this phenomenon and to determine if there were any properties peculiar to eye muscles that differentiated them from ordinary skeletal muscle, the latent period, speed of contraction or rise time, twitch tension, isometric maximal tension, time of relaxation, and finally the relation of initial fiber length to contractile power (length-tension curve) were determined.

The experimental method was to isolate the third nerve, cut it centrally, and sling it across two stimulating electrodes. Monopolar recording electrodes were generally used, placed on the muscle and the muscle-tendon junction. The inferior oblique (or occasionally a rectus muscle) was attached to an isometric strain gauge by a short length of stiff, fine wire hooked into the tendon. The recording was made after appropriate amplification and photographed on a double-beam oscilloscope.

All measurements of extraocular muscle tension were made using strain gauges with linear outputs of 0 to 140 Gm. Measurements of limb skeletal muscle were made with heavier gauges of up to 10 Kg. or by attaching to the tendon a heavy spring steel lever for greater forces. The techniques of the various experimental procedures were developed on cats and then repeated on dogs.

Variation in stimulus voltage, pulse duration, or repetition rate

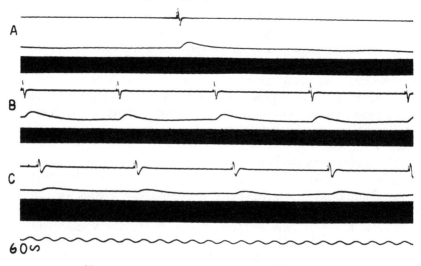

FIGURE 63. ACTION POTENTIAL AND ISOMETRIC TWITCH CONTRACTION

Cat inferior oblique muscle; bipolar recording electrodes and strain gauge tension measurements. A, example of average twitch response to a single supramaximal stimulus to motor nerve; B, after moderate tetanic stimulation to produce beginning signs of fatigue; C, after severe tetanic stimulation to produce marked fatigue and contracture. (Time = 60 cycles per sec.)

elicited only the responses typical of skeletal muscle. Activation of low-threshold, large-diameter nerve fibers with minimal stimulus voltage, as well as activation of relatively small diameter fibers through anodal polarization or compression blocks, produced only changes in muscle contraction amplitude.

The smooth, fast rise and decay times of the twitch contraction in ocular muscle of the cat were within the reported range of 7–9 msec. rise and 12–20 msec. decay[51] (Figure 63 A). The diphasic muscle action potential obtained with one electrode placed on the muscle belly and a reference electrode placed at the distal musculotendonous junction, except for amplitude, was unaffected by changes in stimulus voltage or muscle stretch. After repetitive stimulation to produce fatigue and contracture, the records showed only a decrease in tension of the individual twitch contraction; its latency, rise and decay time were relatively unaffected (Figure 63 B). After tetanus, only slight changes in the duration or amplitude of the action potential were detectable until the muscle reached a marked state of fatigue and contracture (Figure 63 C). Repetitive nerve stimulation with muscle stretch brought about an increase in amplitude of the first few action potentials, the stretch effect (Figure 64).

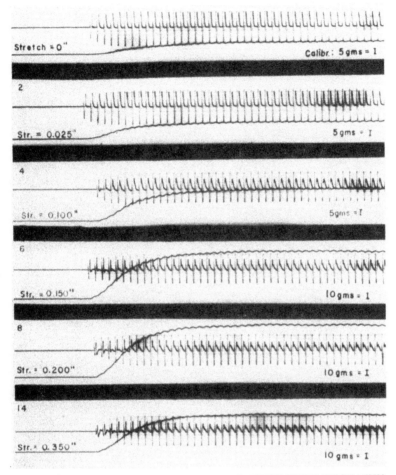

FIGURE 64. CAT RIGHT LATERAL RECTUS MUSCLE, DIRECT NERVE STIMULATION
Upper beam, EMG bipolar electrode recording; *lower beam,* strain gauge
tension. Traces 2, 4, 6, 8, increasing contractile power with increasing
initial length (stretch). Trace 14, decreased strength of contraction with
excesive stretch.

We did not observe any secondary, slower action potential wave
succeeding the main action potential by increasing the strength of
stimulation as reported by Brown and Harvey.[42] All fibers responded
with little temporal dispersion even during the continual depression
or suppression of neuromuscular transmission with atropine and succinylcholine. The positive after-potential following the spike was
suspected (by Brown and Harvey) of possibly being due to the monopolar method of recording. However, the positive after-potential is

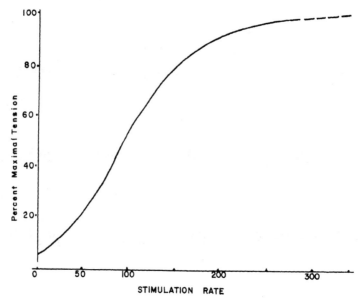

STIMULATION RATE

FIGURE 65. CAT INFERIOR OBLIQUE MUSCLE, DIRECT NERVE STIMULATION;
EFFECT OF STIMULATION FREQUENCY ON STRENGTH OF CONTRACTION

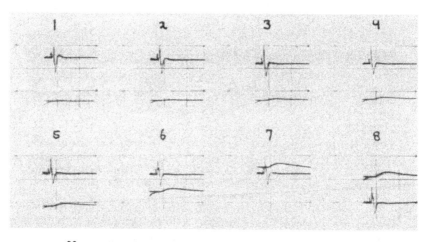

FIGURE 66. CAT INFERIOR OBLIQUE MUSCLE; OSCILLOSCOPE PHOTOGRAPHS DEPICTING
EFFECT OF SINGLE SHOCK STIMULUS TO INFERIOR OBLIQUE NERVE

Upper trace, small artifact followed by diphasic muscle action potential; *lower
trace,* strain gauge tension. Numbers 1–8, increasing muscle stretch with no
effect on action potential; number 3, perceptible twitch tension developing;
numbers 2–8, highest twitch tension develops after 3 Gm. stretch tension.

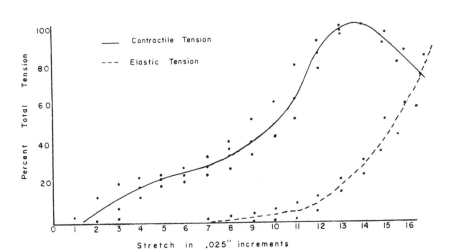

FIGURE 67. CAT INFERIOR OBLIQUE MUSCLE, DIRECT NERVE STIMULATION
Length-tension curves from three preparations, indicating tetanic contractile force
with 0.025 inch increments of stretch.

also recorded by a concentric needle electrode and can be potentiated by repetition, and it was concluded that it must therefore be a phenomenon of muscle repolarization.

It was found that a relatively smooth tetanic contraction did not occur until about 200 stimuli or more per minute were delivered (Figure 65). Even at higher rates of stimulation, contraction and relaxation time are so fast in the inferior oblique muscle of the cat that it can still respond with a slight increase in tension to each stimulus. This is in contrast to peripheral limb muscle.

The length-tension relation was plotted from the weight-calibrated strain gauge for either twitch tension (Figure 66) or tetanic tension (Figure 64) on the oscilloscope and ink writer. The tension developed was plotted in increments of 0.025 inch of stretch from the maximally shortened state below rest length to that where the elastic tension was greater than the contractile strength.

The elastic tension was found to exhibit an exponential increase with stretch while the contractile power developed tension in a more linear fashion over that portion of stretch which was calculated to be within or close to the physiological range of passive tension as measured with an intact globe. With passive tension above and below this range contractile power decreased (Figure 67).

Contractile tension measurements made at moderate stretch tensions were repeatable in the same preparation. Those measurements made with high degrees of stretch, at or beyond the point where stretch tension equalled or exceeded contractile power, were not. Measurements of contractile power after excessive stretch were found to be greater at low stretch tensions, but exhibited a decrease of 50 percent or more in maximal contractile strength. The elastic tension, however, was relatively unaffected.

Within the physiological range neither the elastic tension nor muscle length had an appreciable effect on the ability of the muscle to follow high rates of stimulation, nor did it appear to alter its fusion frequency. Also the rise time for maximal tension development at any length in this range was relatively unaffected (Figure 64).

After fusion frequency of stimulation with the muscle at resting length, a 10-fold or more increase in contractile tension was obtained by stretching the muscle to optimal length (Figure 64).

In a sample experiment it was found that with about 0.4 in. of stretch above the completely relaxed (tendon cut) position, the muscle was under approximately 1 Gm. of elastic tension and produced a total of almost 14 Gm. of contractile tension when stimulated maximally at 150–200 per sec.

The maximal power of contraction fell off quickly with stretch above 5 Gm. of elastic tension. The elastic tension quickly exceeded developed contractile force with slight increments of stretch. On the other hand, about one gram of stretch tension had to be applied before the muscle could develop any appreciable contractile power.

Conclusions: Stretch-Tension Relationship.–

1. There is a similar relation of tension produced by active contraction and stretch tension in extraocular and limb skeletal muscle.

2. There is no evidence for a smooth muscle contractile mechanism in extraocular muscle.

3. Maximal tension is obtained only after a certain degree of stretch.

4. Small increments of stretch have large effects on the muscle contractile power.

5. Muscle efficiency is greatest over a specific interval of length and elastic tension.

6. Excessive tension produces a decrease in muscle power.

7. The same values of contractile and elastic tension are found after repeated moderate muscle stretch. After excessive stretch the elastic tension values are replicable, the contractile tension values are not.

INNERVATION AND MUSCLE TENSION. In the nerve-muscle preparation, tension is a function of frequency. Lippold[93] has shown that a linear relation exists between the integrated electromyogram and tension in voluntary isometric contraction. No proportion was found between mechanical and electric responses of a single motor unit, but when the summated effect of a large number of units was recorded the variations statistically canceled out. He assumed that recruitment must be random. This relation was also shown in the nerve muscle preparation by Bigland, Hutter, and Lippold[12] and in fatigue.[63]

Kuboki[88] reported the irregularity in discharge pattern of single motor units at certain frequencies and the lack of relationship existing between the activity of individual units and ocular movement; although, in general, units were noted to increase their frequency in accordance with the movement. It would appear unwise, therefore, to expect the correlation of single unit discharges with muscle tension, but the over-all sampling of the muscle does reflect a significant relationship of frequency to movement.[37]

Bigland and Lippold,[13] in 1954, found a direct proportion between integrated electric activity and tension during constant velocity of shortening or lengthening and a linear relation between tension and the number and frequency of units. Inman and associates[76] found a linear relation between electric integral and tension in isometric contraction with monopolar surface and coaxial electrodes, but no quantitative relation when the muscle was permitted to change in length.

The electric integral obtained in extraocular muscle *in situ* is recorded under isotonic, not isometric, conditions. Hence, it becomes a problem to determine whether the integral bears a true linear relationship to the muscle tension or not. An approach to these problems in man and experimental animals has been developed, employing the strain gauge technique.[40,41]

It is important in assaying electric activity of muscle that a representative sampling area be obtained. Monopolar electrodes are capable of a wide-range pickup; the coaxial or concentric electrodes have a more restricted pickup. The type of electrode, at least in peripheral skeletal muscle, did not seem to make much difference in the recording of electric integrals.[76] The finer concentric electrodes (30 gauge) have been best suited for this purpose in extraocular muscle.[40,41]

In studies on the integrated electric activity of extraocular muscle, Momosse stated that the relation between tension and integral was linear at a constant velocity of shortening and lengthening, the gradient of the line being less in lengthening.[109] Such a relationship had also been shown in peripheral skeletal muscle.[13]

Momosse's figures demonstrated smooth curves of electric integral compared with the position of the eye, with a steeper ascendancy as one entered more into the field of action of the tested muscle. Relaxation showed a similar curve but at a slightly lower level. The more the velocity of shortening increased, the more linear became the shortening integral. The lengthening curve, however, appeared relatively constant. These relationships were quite similar in extraocular muscle and peripheral skeletal muscle.

Breinin[37] showed a similar linearity of vertical and horizontal muscles, employing a different technique of integration. It seems a reasonable assumption that the movement of the globe can be equated with muscle tension since such movement is a reflection of the preponderating influence and tension of the agonist. Using a pulse count technique based upon differentiation of motor units, Breinin[37] showed that a fair degree of linearity exists in ocular movement versus frequency with a marked fall-off in the number of pulses at the extreme limit of the fixational field. This paralleled the phenomenon observed with integration. The fall-off may be due to electrode displacement, although it has also been attributed to inhibition.[110] The pulse count of a muscle in movement out of its field of action may in some sampling areas reveal a stepwise decrease.

The foregoing studies suggest that even in the isotonic contraction of extraocular muscle in man the electric integral and frequency bear a reasonably linear relationship to tension.

In cats, the experimental determination of length-tension curves for nerve-muscle preparations of the inferior oblique (either twitch or tetanus) showed that with a constant-amplitude stimulus the strength of contraction is proportional to the initial length of the muscle.[40] Thus, with a constant stimulus, a stretched extraocular muscle produces a much larger rise in tension than does a shortened muscle. This tension rise increases with initial length up to a critical point, after which the tension falls off rapidly. In this behavior the extraocular muscles are entirely similar to peripheral skeletal muscle.

It follows that the low-level electric activity of the stretched extraocular muscle out of its field of action is adequate to produce sufficient tension to cause rotation. With progressive contraction of the muscle as it rotates into its field of action, a greater innervation is required to elicit comparable amounts of tension. At the most extreme limit of its field of action the largest amount of electric activity cannot elicit any further tension increase or additional rotation. Indeed, a greater effort of innervation may only succeed in producing a deficit of rotation.

In another direct approach to muscle tension, Madroszkiewicz[96] measured the strength of extraocular muscle with an ophthalmodynamometer at surgery in normal and strabismus patients. The maximum strength of a medial rectus was recorded as 61 Gm. In convergent squint the medial rectus strength predominated over the lateral rectus. In divergent strabismus the lateral rectus muscle predominated. In general, however, the difference in muscle strength was only a few grams. In paralytic squint the ocular muscle exhibited very little or no power. In the normal eye the strength of the horizontal recti muscles appeared equal, and each was able to carry a weight of about 60 Gm.

The combined electromyogram and strain gauge technique in man should help to resolve many of the controversial problems of extraocular muscle physiology. Tension, the most important resultant of electric activity, can be determined without the possibility of confusion due to electric artifacts. Unfortunately, as yet, this technique in man can be applied only during surgical procedures.

TONIC ACTIVITY. A high level of spontaneous activity in extraocular muscle can be furnished by the bulbar reticular activating system. This is seen by recording the extraocular electromyogram in the decerebrate and spinally transected cat. After the anesthetic wears off, if the cat is comfortable and the room fairly quiet, it may appear to sleep. Little or no electric activity may be recorded from the electrodes implanted in the extraocular muscles. A loud whistle or a pinch on the ear can arouse the cat. This is signaled by EEG changes, lid opening, and subsequent eye movement. Recordings at this time generally show a fairly rapid onset of electric activity in the ocular muscle which may reach a maximal level. After a short time the activity decays to the former state. The experiment can be repeated many times. A similar arousal sequence of extraocular muscle activity in humans recovering from general anesthesia and awakening from sleep has been electromyographically recorded.[33]

The spontaneous electric activity is dependent not only upon intact innervation from the brain stem but also in part upon a certain degree of stretch tension. Like peripheral skeletal muscle the extraocular muscle is electrically silent when its central nervous system connection is severed. Tension recorded under these conditions is passive and due to the elastic fiber component. Spontaneous electric activity may also be obliterated in the lightly anesthetized or decerebrate cat when the extraocular muscle is freed from the globe and surrounding connective tissue and allowed to recoil upon itself inside the orbital cavity. Spontaneous activity may be recorded again when the muscle is stretched.

The continuous activity so characteristic of extraocular muscles in conscious animals and man appears intimately related to the reticular activating system, modified to some extent by feedback from the muscles themselves. Indeed, this may be one of the disputed functions of the ocular muscle spindles and other receptors with their central connections.

The constant activity of extraocular muscle in the primary position must greatly facilitate the remarkable speed, precision, and coordination of eye movements since slack is taken up and jerkiness is minimized.

Although the principle of reciprocal innervation was described by Sherrington on the basis of ocular muscle studies, a true ocular myotatic (stretch) reflex as found in limb skeletal muscle is not present in animals or man.[30,71,101] Sudden stretch of an ocular muscle may produce no response or a cocontraction of several ocular muscles of the same or opposite eye. McCouch and Adler[101] believed this reaction in the cat to be a withdrawal reflex since it was chiefly noted in the retractor bulbi muscles. We have observed that sudden stretch may produce in agonist and antagonist an increase in tension but not the fast, monosynaptic response as found in limb skeletal muscle.[40] No inhibitory responses to stretch such as have been reported in man[122] were noted. Indeed the muscles of the opposite eye may also show an increase in tension and the intact globe may be observed to retract slightly. A similar response was also obtained in some instances with stimulation of the central stump of the nerve to the extraocular muscle. Stimulation in these experiments did not produce a relaxation of antagonist muscles in the same or opposite eye as one might expect on the basis of reciprocal inhibition. Instead of a decrease in spontaneous activity, there was in some instances a general increase. This increase in activity was indistinguishable from reticular arousal.

In view of the finding of extraocular muscle spindles in man and many animal species,[50] the recording of afferent activity with stretch,[52] the presence of gamma efferents,[144] and since stretch of ocular muscle in man is not necessarily painful, there seems little doubt that feedback from extraocular muscle subserves more than a simple nociceptive reflex response.

QUANTITATION OF INNERVATION (SEE FIGURES 68 TO 72)

The necessity for quantitative techniques in assessing innervation in the extraocular muscles became apparent quite early, since kinesiology is such an important aspect of their physiology.[31,37,38] The inspection of the electromyogram itself is a very inadequate method of

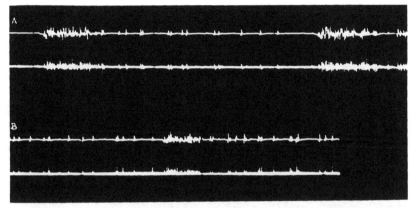

FIGURE 68. ELECTROMYOGRAM OF INFERIOR OBLIQUE AND DIFFERENTIAL
Upper trace, signal; *lower trace*, differential. A, biphasic; B, positive polarity.

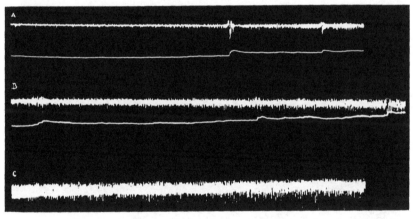

FIGURE 69. ELECTROMYOGRAM OF INFERIOR OBLIQUE IN GAZE DOWN TO UP
Continuous integrator, *lower trace*.

determining the level of activity since frequency, amplitude, and the number of potentials all contribute to the electric sum of activity. It is extremely difficult to assess these various factors properly by visual methods. This is a general problem in neuromuscular electrophysiology and has resulted in the development of electronic integrators which accomplish the summing up of the total energy developed at any given moment.[31,59,76,109] This sum is then displayed in some readily identifiable form. Various types of integrators have been devised based upon amplitude or frequency displays. Breinin[31] used an amplitude display

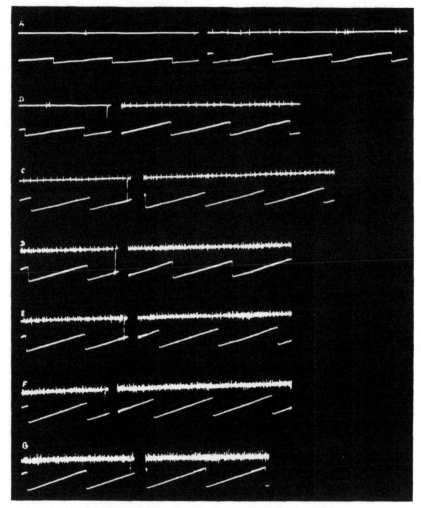

FIGURE 70. ELECTROMYOGRAM OF INFERIOR OBLIQUE
—40 to +30 degrees—depression to elevation. Integrator, *lower trace.*

of a capacitor discharging at regularly selected intervals in the form
of a saw-tooth wave. The height of the vertical component of the wave
is proportional to the electric integral. One can then determine the
sum of activity by measuring this vertical discharge line with a
straight edge. Momosse[109] used a continuous integrator in which the
electric integral was actually an average-amplitude display closely
following the average energy of the input signal. The former method

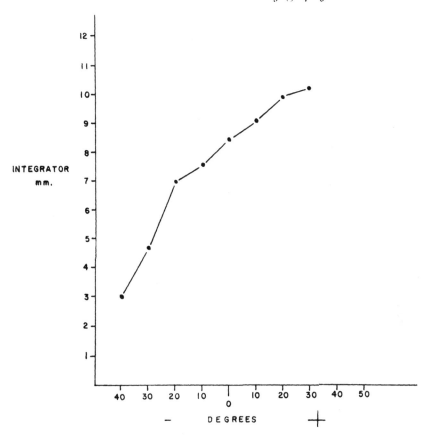

FIGURE 71. GRAPH OF INTEGRATOR MEASUREMENTS OF INFERIOR OBLIQUE
−40 to +30 degrees.

has the advantage of ready mensuration and does not require co-ordinates. The latter provides a very simple comparison but requires coordinates for measurement. Each has its virtues and failings, but either method can be used advantageously in assessing muscle activity.

Breinin[37] employed a different technique to correlate frequency of firing with activity of the muscle. In this system, motor units are differentiated to form a population of pulses. A pulse is generated for each major slope change in the signal. In this way, overlapping units which are not perfectly synchronized will generate spikes, thus re-vealing the presence of multiple units. A discriminating adjustment permits the differentiation of units of selected amplitude. By means of a diode the signal can be converted into either positive or negative

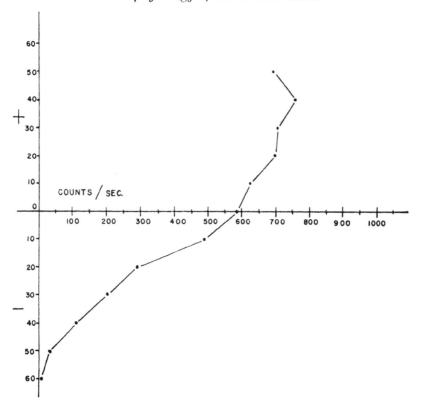

FIGURE 72. GRAPH OF LEFT INFERIOR OBLIQUE FREQUENCY IN MOVEMENT: DOWN
TO UP

output polarity. The population of spikes obtained appears on a stable
base line that is independent of movement artifacts in the signal. The
time constants of the differentiator sort out all low-frequency interference, allowing only the essentially high-frequency motor units to
pass through. The spikes are then processed through an electronic
counter which prints out the total number as a digital record. Such
data can then be handled readily in statistical fashion. In addition,
one may readily make an analog record of the same data with a
potentiometer or galvanometer recorder. Differentiation does not
reflect total electric activity; it simply records pulse rates. It has already
been pointed out that the pulse rate bears a useful relationship to
tension. During constant fixation, pulse counts produce reliable, reproducible correlations. Variations occur during movement of the eye,

but it is possible to obtain consistent counts demonstrating a good degree of linearity. The combination of integrating and differentiating techniques may be considered a calculus of muscle activity. The combination permits a high degree of quantitation of the electric activity in muscle. This is important in kinesiologic studies and in pathologic states such as myasthenia where one can readily see the quantitative loss of activity in the myasthenic reaction and the recovery of activity through rest or drugs (Table 1).

TABLE 1. MYASTHENIA GRAVIS: DIFFERENTIAL PULSE COUNT RESPONSE OF OCULAR MUSCLE TO EDROPHONIUM

After 90 sec.	After 1 min.	
−00003	−00258	00790
00006	00162	00802
00008	00246	00775
00133	00325	00791
00225	00327	00729
00238	00364	00644
00157	00382	00641
00147	00409	00637
00128	00447	00489
00232	00516	00435
00194	00607	00328
00196	00603	00285
00225	00638	00161
00233	00749	00099
	00771	00007

Tensilon I. V.: −00007
Base line: −00000

Pulse height analysis[41] is particularly revealing in automatically demonstrating amplitude variations in normal and disordered muscle. Pulse height analysis is performed by an Elex model 101 B5 channel analyzer. Pulses may be sorted and counted in five separate categories dependent only on their maximum amplitude. The channel separation and lower starting point are adjustable allowing different amplitude spreads to be handled and noise near the base line to be ignored. The instrument includes such provisions as remote start-stop, counting all pulses above the top channel if desired, and use as a conventional counter.

In addition to these techniques, Breinin[41] is employing spectrum analysis to demonstrate the Fourier frequency content of the electric signal in extraocular muscle.

Such studies may prove of considerable clinical value in differentiating the myopathic process at an earlier stage than can be accomplished by any other technique. It has been noted that myopathy in
its early stages even in the presence of marked palsies may exhibit
electric activity visibly indistinguishable from the normal. It is hoped
that a certain proportion of these can be diagnosed through frequency
analysis since the mean duration of myopathic units is less than of
normal units.[41]

It is of interest that some cases of myasthenia gravis also show
elements of the myopathic response. The spectrum analysis technique
which was reported by Walton[140] for peripheral skeletal muscle may
prove equally valuable in the study of extraocular muscle.

APPRAISAL OF OCULAR ELECTROMYOGRAPHY

It has been repeatedly pointed out that electromyography is an invaluable research tool and in the case of the extraocular muscles is
proving of great interest and service in determining normal physiology.
Its use in muscular problems of children is extremely limited because
of the restricted application of the technique in children. This does
not mean that children cannot be examined by electromyography but
that considerable selectivity is necessary. In favorable cases one may
carry out very adequate electromyographic studies.

In general, comitant strabismus does not require electromyography,
since one does not encounter abnormalities in the electric firing of
muscle. Certain kinds of strabismus, however, are decidedly suitable
for electromyographic investigation. These include the pseudopalsies,
such as the superior oblique sheath syndrome, Duane's syndrome, and
blowout fracture of the orbit. The primary application of electromyography, however, is in the field of neurologic disturbances. All types
of paretic strabismus are candidates for electromyography. Palsies must
be of moderate or severe degree to demonstrate electromyographic
changes. Where full rotations are still possible, there is little point
in carrying out an electromyographic investigation. Myasthenia gravis
is perhaps the most important indication for ocular electromyography.
The diagnosis can be made in many individuals in whom clinical
evidences are borderline in character. Myopathies can be diagnosed
and, in fact, may became evident where they were least suspected.
The prognosis of a lesion may be estimated by the presence and
character of electric activity and the extent of palsies determined.
The possibilities inherent in this technique are very great.

Criticisms of the role of electromyography in strabismus[133] are ill founded since there is abundant evidence that such investigations may clarify many obscure affections of the extraocular muscles and may reveal unexpected involvements in others. There are many potential sources of error in electromyography based upon instrumentation, technique, or interpretation. The steadily swelling body of evidence should clarify legitimate electric patterns and their relationship to the physiology of normal and disordered extraocular muscle. In all such investigations, scientific interest must be tempered with good judgment. Scientifically important observations may be achieved with a minimum of electrode insertions. Ocular electromyography has already proved itself as a most important diagnostic modality in the study of neuromuscular disease. As a research tool it is providing great advances in the understanding of the role of innervation in the physiology of extraocular muscle.

On the basis of this survey of electrophysiology of the extraocular muscles, it becomes evident that there is a fundamental kinship between extraocular and peripheral skeletal muscle in which similarities far exceed the differences. Although the literature is replete with references to the uniqueness of extraocular muscle, the evidence does not support this conclusion. The structural, physiologic, and pharmacologic differences which exist are quantitative rather than qualitative and may be viewed as adaptations to the highly specialized role of extraocular muscle. Both types of muscle obey similar laws, exhibit similar properties, and react similarly to disease. The classical principles of neuromuscular physiology apply equally to both.

REFERENCES

1. Adler, F. H., Pathologic physiology of strabismus, A.M.A. Arch. Ophth., 50:19–29, 1953.
2. Adrian, E. D., and D. W. Bronk, Discharge of impulses in motor nerve fibers; frequency of discharge in reflex and voluntary contractions, J. Physiol., 67:119–151, 1929.
3. Alpern, M., and P. Ellen, A quantitative analysis of the horizontal movements of the eyes in the experiments of Johannes Mueller, 1 and 2, Am. J. Ophth., 42 (Pt. 2):289–301, 1956.
4. Alpern, M., and J. Wolter, The relation of horizontal saccadic and vergence movements, A.M.A. Arch. Ophth., 56:685–690, 1956.
5. Alpern, M., Discussion of Tamler, Jampolsky, and Marg, 1958.
6. Ambrosio, A.; A. Barone; and C. Serra, Prime osservazioni sull'attivita elettrica dei muscoli oculari estrinseci durante la stimolazione luminosa intermittente, Boll. Soc. Ital. Biol. Sper., 33:1218–1221, 1957.
7. Ambrosio, A., and M. D'Esposito, Sindrome di Turk-Duane, contributo clinico ed elettromiografico, Arch. Ottal., 299:7, 1957.
8. Barone, A., and C. Serra, Risposta dell'effettore muscolare all stimulazione luminosa intermittente, Boll. Soc. Ital. Biol. Sper., 33:1216–1218, 1957.
9. Bartels, M., Ueber Regulierung des Augenstellung durch den Ohrapparat III, von Graefes Arch. Ophth., 78:129–182, 1911.
10. Bartels, M., Ueber willkürliche und unwillkürliche Augenbewegungen (Nystagmus der blinden, proprioreflexe Blickbewegungen der Tiere), Klin. Mbl. Augenheilk., 53:358–370, 1914.
11. Bender, M. B., and J. R. Fulton, Factors in functional recovery following section of oculomotor nerve in monkeys, J. Neurol. & Psychol., 2:285–292, 1939.
12. Bigland, B.; O. F. Hutter; and O. C. J. Lippold, Action potentials and tension in nerve muscle preparations, J. Physiol., 121:55P., 1953.
13. Bigland, B., and O. C. J. Lippold, Relation between force, velocity and integrated electrical activity in human muscles, J. Physiol., 123:214–224, 1954.
14. Bjork, A., Electrical activity of human extrinsic eye muscles, Experientia, 8:226–227, 1952.
15. Bjork, A., and E. Kugelberg, Motor unit activity in the human extraocular muscles, Electroencephalog. & Clin. Neurophysiol., 5:271–278, 1953.
16. Bjork, A., and E. Kugelberg, The electrical activity of the muscles of the eye and eyelids in various positions and during movement, Electroencelphalog. & Clin. Neurophysiol., 5:595–602, 1953.
17. Bjork, A., Electromyographic study of conditions involving limited mobility of the eye chiefly due to neurogenic pareses, Brit. J. Ophth., 38:528–544, 1954.
18. Bjork, A., Electromyographic studies on the coordination of antagonistic muscles in cases of abducens and facial palsy, Brit. J. Ophth., 38:605–615, 1954.

19. Bjork, A., The electromyogram of the extraocular muscles in opticokinetic nystagmus and in reading, Acta Ophth., 33:437–454, 1955.

20. Bjork, A.; M. Halldin; and A. Wahlin, Enophthalmos elicited by succinylcholine: Some observations on the effect of succinylcholine and noradrenaline on the intraorbital muscles studied on man and experimental animals, Acta Anesth. Scand., 1:41–53, 1957.

21. Blodi, F. C., and M. W. Van Allen, Electromyography of extraocular muscles in fusional movements: 1, Electric phenomena at the breakpoint of fusion, Am. J. Ophth., 44:136–142, 1957.

22. Blodi, F. C., Discussion of Tamler, Jampolsky, and Marg, 1958.

23. Bornschein, H., and G. Schubert, Elektromyographie des Drehnystagmus, Wien. Ztschr. Nervenh., 5:149–154, 1952.

24. Bors, E., Ueber das Zahlenverhältnis zwischen Nerven und Muskelfasern, Anat. Anzeiger, 60:415–416, 1925–6.

25. Brecher, G. A., and W. G. Mitchell, Studies on the role of sympathetic nervous stimulation in extraocular muscle movements, Am. J. Ophth., 44 (Pt. 2): 144–149, 1957.

26. Breinin, G. M., and J. Moldaver, Electromyography of the human extraocular muscles: 1, Normal kinesiology: divergence mechanism, A.M.A. Arch. Ophth., 54:200–210, 1955.

27. Breinin, G. M., The nature of vergence revealed by electromyography, A.M.A. Arch. Ophth., 54:407–409, 1955.

28. Breinin, G. M., Electromyography—a tool in ocular and neurologic diagnosis: I, Myasthenia gravis, A.M.A. Arch. Ophth., 57:161–164, 1957.

29. Breinin, G. M., Electromyography—a tool in ocular and neurologic diagnosis: II, Muscle palsies, A.M.A. Arch. Ophth., 57:165–175, 1957.

30. Breinin, G. M., Electromyographic evidence for ocular muscle proprioception in man, A.M.A. Arch. Ophth., 57:176–180, 1957.

31. Breinin, G. M., Quantitation of extraocular muscle innervation, A.M.A. Arch. Ophth., 57:644–650, 1957.

32. Breinin, G. M., Electrophysiologic insight in ocular motility, Am. Orthopt. J., 7:5–19, 1957.

33. Breinin, G. M., The position of rest during anesthesia and sleep: Electromyographic observations, A.M.A. Arch. Ophth., 57:323–326, 1957.

34. Breinin, G. M., New aspects of ophthalmoneurologic diagnosis, A.M.A. Arch. Ophth., 58:375–388, 1957.

35. Breinin, G. M., The nature of vergence revealed by electromyography: II, Accommodative and fusional vergence, A.M.A. Arch. Ophth., 58:623–631, 1957.

36. Breinin, G. M., Electromyography—a tool in ocular and neurologic diagnosis: III, Supranuclear mechanisms, A.M.A. Arch. Ophth., 59:177–187, 1958.

37. Breinin, G. M., Analytic studies of the electromyogram of human extraocular muscle, Am. J. Ophth., 46 (Pt. 2):123–142, 1958.

38. Breinin, G. M., Quantitative electronic techniques in ocular motility, Tr. N. Y. Acad. Sci., Ser. 2, 21:605–608, 1959.

39. Breinin, G. M., Contributions of electromyography to strabismus (Holmes memorial lecture), Proc. Inst. Med. Chicago, 22:303–309, 1959.

40. Breinin, G. M., and J. Perryman, Unpublished observations.

41. Breinin, G. M., Unpublished observations.

42. Brown, G. L., and A. M. Harvey, Neuromuscular transmission in the extrinsic muscles of the eye, J. Physiol., 99:379–399, 1941.

43. Buchthal, F., An Introduction to Electromyography. Copenhagen, Gyldendal, 1957.

44. Charnwood, J., Proprioception in the extraocular muscles, Optical Developments, 24, no. 1, Rochester, N.Y., Bausch and Lomb Opt. Co., January 1954. (*Also* Optics, no. 103, Scotland, July 1951.)

45. Cilimbaris, P. A., Histologische Untersuchungen über die Muskelspindeln der Augenmuskeln, Arch. f. Mikr. Anat., 75:692–747, 1910.

46. Clark, D. A., Muscle counts of motor units: A study in innervation ratios, Am. J. Physiol., 96:296–304, 1931.

47. Cogan, D. G., Neurology of the Ocular Muscles, 2nd ed., Springfield, Ill., Charles C. Thomas, 1956, p. 103.

48. Cooper, S., and P. M. Daniel, Muscle spindles in human extrinsic eye muscles, Brain, 72:1–24, 1949.

49. Cooper, S., and P. M. Daniel, Responses from the stretch receptors of the goat's extrinsic eye muscles with an intact motor innervation, Quart. J. Exper. Physiol., 42:222–231, 1957.

50. Cooper, S.; P. M. Daniel; and D. Whitteridge, Muscle spindles and other sensory endings in the extrinsic eye muscles: The physiology and anatomy of these receptors and their connections with the brainstem, Brain, 78:564, 1955.

51. Cooper, S., and J. C. Eccles, The isometric responses of mammalian muscles, J. Physiol., 69:377–385, 1930.

52. Cooper, S., and J. Fillenz, Afferent discharge in response to stretch from the extraocular muscles of cat and monkey and the innervation of these muscles, J. Physiol., 127:400–413, 1955.

53. de Kleyn, A., Ueber vestibulare Augen-reflexe: IV, Experimentelle Untersuchungen über die schnelle Phase des vestibularen Nystagmus beim Kaninchen, von Graefes Arch. Ophth., 107:480–488, 1922.

54. Denny-Brown, D., Interpretation of the electromyogram, Arch. Neurol. & Psychiat., 6:99, 1949.

55. Denny-Brown, D., and J. Pennybacker, Fibrillation and fasciculation in voluntary muscle, Brain, 61:311–334, 1938.

56. D'Esposito, M.; C. Serra; and A. Ambrosio, Acquisizioni recente in neuroftalmologia: La'Elettromiografia dei muscoli oculari, Arch. Ottal., 63:183–210, 1959.

57. Dillon, J. B.; P. Sabawala; D. B. Taylor; and R. Gunter, Action of succinylcholine on extraocular muscles and intraocular pressure, Anesthesiology, 18:44–49, 1957.

58. Dreyfus, P. M.; S. Hakim; and R. D. Adams, Diabetic ophthalmoplegia, A.M.A. Arch. Neurol. Psychiat., 77:337–349, 1957.

59. Drohocki, Z., An electronic integrator for the automatic measurements of average tension in the electroencephalogram, Electroencephalog. & Clin. Neurophysiol., 8:706–707, 1956.

60. Dubois-Reymond, E., Untersuchungen über Thierische Elektrizität. Berlin, G. Reimer, 1948.

61. Duke-Elder, W. S., and P. M. Duke-Elder, The contraction of the extrinsic muscles of the eye by choline and nicotine, Proc. Roy. Soc., B, 107:332–343, 1930.

62. Eaton, L. M., and E. H. Lambert, Electromyography and electric stimulation of nerves in diseases of motor unit: Observations on myasthenic syndrome associated with malignant tumours, J.A.M.A., 163:1117–1124, 1957.

63. Edwards, R. G., and O. C. J. Lippold, The relation between force and integrated activity in fatigued muscle, J. Physiol., 132:677–681, 1956.

64. Erlanger, J., Analysis of the action potential in nerve, Harvey Lect. 22:90–113, 1926.

65. Erlanger, J., and W. Gasser, Electrical Signs of Nervous Activity. Philadelphia, University of Pennsylvania Press, 1937.
66. Esslen, E.; H. G. Mertens; and W. Papst, Die ocularen Myopathien: I. Report, Nervenarzt, 29:10–16, 1958. Die chronische okulare Myositis: II. Report, Nervenarzt, 29:120–127, 1958.
67. Glees, M., Eine Methode zur Elektromyographie der Augenmuskeln, Ber. deutsch. ophth. Gesellsch., 58:307–310, 1953.
68. Gordon, G., Observations upon the movements of the eyelids, Brit. J. Ophth., 35:339–351, 1951.
69. Hering, E., Beiträge zur allgemeinen Nerven und Muskelphysiologie, Sitzungsb. Akad. Wissensch. Math-naturw. Cl., Wien, 79:137, 1879.
70. Hoffmann, P., Ueber die Aktionsströme der Augenmuskeln bei Ruhe des Tieres und beim Nystagmus, Arch. f. Anat. u. Physiol., 37:23–34, 1913.
71. Hoffmann, P., Ist es möglich die physiologischen Erfahrungen über die Sehnenreflexe (Eigenreflexe) mit den Pathologischen in Einklang zu bringen? Nervenarzt, 2:641–656, 1929.
72. Hofmann, H., and H. Holzer, Die Wirkung von Muskelrelaxantien auf den intraokularen Druck, Klin. Mbl. Augenheilk., 123:1–16, 1953.
73. Hofmann, H., and F. Lembeck, Das Verhalten der äusseren Augenmuskeln gegenüber Curare, Dekamethonium (ClO), und Succinylcholin (M115), Arch. Exper. Path. u. Pharmakol., 216:552–557, 1952.
74. Huber, A., and F. H. Lehner, Zur Elektromyographie der Augenmuskeln, Ophth., 131:238–247, 1956.
75. Huber, A., Myasthenia (maladie de Erb-Goldflam) et paralysies des muscles oculaires, Bull. et mem. Soc. Franc. Opht., 70:216–228, 1957.
76. Inman, V. T.; H. J. Ralston; J. B. Saunders; B. Feinstein; and E. Wright, Relation of human electromyogram to muscular tension, Electroencephalog. & Clin. Neurophysiol., 4:187–194, 1952.
77. Jampolsky, A.; E. Tamler; and E. Marg, Artifacts and normal variations in human ocular electromyography, A.M.A. Arch. Ophth., 61:402–413, 1959.
78. Kamouchi, T., Electromyographic study in neurogenic palsy of extraocular and levator muscles, Acta Soc. Ophth. Jap., 59:791–803, 1955. *Also* Jap. J. Ophth., 1:30–34, 1957.
79. Kamouchi, T., Electromyographic studies on extraocular and levator palpebrae muscles: Time series analysis of current discharge interval of single N.M.U. spikes, Acta Soc. Ophth. Jap., 60:1675–1686, 1956.
80. Kamouchi, T., Electromyographic studies on the extraocular muscles: About the influence of flicker stimulation on the current discharge interval of single N.M.U. spike and its time series analysis results, Acta Soc. Ophth. Jap., 61:943–950, 1957.
81. Kollner, H., and P. Hoffmann, I, Der Einfluss des vestibular Apparates auf die Innervation der Augenmuskeln, Arch. f. Augenheilk., 90:170–194, 1922.
82. Kollner, H., and P. Hoffmann, Der Einfluss des vestibular Apparates auf die Innervation der Augenmuskeln: 2, Galvanischer Nystagmus mit willkürlicher Frequenz und die Innervationsverhältnisse in den zentralen Nervenbahnen, Arch. f. Augenheilk., 92:272–281, 1923.
83. Kornblueth, W.; A. Jampolsky; E. Tamler; and E. Marg, Activity of the oculorotary muscles during tonometry and tonography: An electromyographic study, A.M.A. Arch. Ophth., 62:555–561, 1959.
84. Kuboki, T., Electromyogram of the extrinsic eye muscles of man, Acta Soc. Ophth. Jap., 58:874–877, 1954.
85. Kuboki, T., The electromyogram of the extrinsic eye muscles of man: Second report, Acta Soc. Ophth. Jap., 59:530–538, 1955.

86. Kuboki, T., Electromyograph of human extraocular muscles: III, During slow movements of the eye, Acta Soc. Ophth. Jap., 60:29–37, 1956.

87. Kuboki, T., Studies of discharge intervals of a single motor unit in the human extraocular muscles: I, During fixation of the gaze, Tohoku J. Exper. Med., 66:91–96, 1957.

88. Kuboki, T., Studies of discharge intervals of a single motor unit in the human extraocular muscles: II, During horizontal movement of the eye, Tohoku J. Exper. Med., 66:97–105, 1957.

89. Kuboki, T.; I. Sekino; and K. Fukushi, The periodicity in the electromyograph of human extraocular muscles: Report I, Acta Soc. Ophth. Jap., 61:1565–1567, 1958.

90. Kuboki, T.; I. Sekino; A. Tomizawa; S. Mikami; and R. Ogane, The periodicity in the electromyograph of human extraocular muscles: Report II, that of the internal rectus in horizontal positions of the eye, Acta Soc. Ophth. Jap., 62:2361–2366, 1958. *Also* Jap. J. Ophth., 3: 66–74, 1959.

91. Lincoff, H. A.; G. M. Breinin; and A. G. DeVoe, The effect of succinylcholine on the extraocular muscles, Am. J. Ophth., 42:440–444, 1957.

92. Lincoff, H. A.; C. H. Ellis; A. G. DeVoe; E. J. DeBeer; D. J. Impastato; S. Berg; L. Orkin; and H. Magda, The effect of succinylcholine on intraocular pressure, Am. J. Ophth., 40:501–510, 1955.

93. Lippold, O. C. J., Relation between integrated action potentials in human muscle and its isometric tension, J. Physiol., 117:492–499, 1952.

94. Lorente de Nó, R., Observations in nystagmus, Acta Oto. Laryng., 21:416–437, 1935.

95. Lorente de Nó, R., The synaptic delay of the motor neurones, Am. J. Physiol., 111:272–281, 1935.

96. Madroszkiewicz, M., Pomiary sily miesni woczach zezujacych I prawidlowych, Klinika Oczna, 24:255–256, 1954.

97. Magee, A. J., Electromyogram of the extraocular muscles of the rabbit in situ, A.M.A. Arch. Ophth., 52:212–220, 1954.

98. Magee, A. J., The electromyogram of the lateral rectus muscle, Am. J. Ophth., 41:275–285, 1956.

99. Magyar, J.; I. Grosz; and Z. Aszalos, Ocular myopathy (Kiloh-Nevin's disease), Ideggyog Szle, 12:197–203, 1959.

100. Marg, E.; A. Jampolsky; and E. Tamler, Elements of human extraocular electromyography, A.M.A. Arch. Ophth., 61:258–269, 1959.

101. McCouch, G. P., and F. H. Adler, Extraocular reflexes, Am. J. Physiol., 100:78–88, 1932.

102. McIntyre, A. K., The quick component of nystagmus, J. Physiol., 97:8–16, 1939.

103. McLean, J. M., and E. D. W. Norton, Unilateral lid retraction without exophthalmos, A.M.A. Arch. Ophth., 61:681–686, 1959.

104. Mertens, H. G.; E. Esslen; and W. Papst, Die ocularen Myopathien: II. Mitteilung: Die chronische oculare Myositis, Nervenarzt, 29:120–127, 1958.

105. Mertens, H. G.; E. Esslen; and W. Papst, III. Mitteilung: Die oligosymptomatische oculare Myositis (Pseudomyasthenia), Nervenarzt, 29:213–226, 1958.

106. Miller, J., Electromyographic pattern of saccadic eye movements, Am. J. Ophth., 46(Pt. 2):183–186, 1958.

107. Miller, J., The electromyography of vergence movement, A.M.A. Arch. Ophth., 62:790–794, 1959.

108. Moldaver, J., and G. M. Breinin, Electromyography of the extraocular muscles in man, Tr. Am. Neurol., A, 141–144, 1956.

109. Momosse, H., Studies in the action of the extraocular muscles by means of the quantitative measurement of integrated electromyography: Report I, application of integrator and behavior of the horizontal and vertical muscles in monocular movements, Acta Soc. Ophth. Jap., 61:1570–1592, 1957.

110. Momosse, H., Electromyographic studies on the mechanism of limitation of monocular movement, Acta Soc. Ophth. Jap., 62:453–457, 1959. (Jap. J. Ophth. 3:9–13, 1959.)

111. Papst, W.; E. Esslen; and H. G. Mertens, Klinische Erfahrungen mit der Elektromyographie bei ocularen Myopathien, Ber. deutsch. ophth. Gesellsch. Heidelberg, 61:304–308, 1957.

112. Papst, W.; E. Esslen; and H. G. Mertens, Die okulare Muskeldystrophie sog. ophthalmoplegia externa chonica progressiva, Klin. Mbl. Augenheilk., 132:691–707, 1958.

113. Papst, W.; H. G. Mertens; and E. Esslen, Die chronische okulare Myositis: I. Mitteilung: Die exophthalmische okulare Myositis, Klin. Mbl. Augenheilk., 133:673–694, 1958.

114. Papst, W.; H. G. Mertens; and E. Esslen, Die chronische okulare Myositis: II. Mitteilung: Die oligosymptomatische okulare Myositis, Klin. Mbl. Augenheilk., 134:374–396, 1959.

115. Perez-Cirera, R., Untersuchungen über die Aktionsströme der Augenmuskeln, Arch. f. Augenheilk., 105:453–459, 1932.

116. Piper, H., Ueber den willkürlichen Muskeltetanus, Arch. ges. Physiol., 119: 301–338, 1907.

117. Piper, H., Elektrophysiologie der Menschlichen Muskeln. Berlin, Julius Springer, 1912.

118. Pulfrich, K., Aktionsströme äusserer Augenmuskeln (einschliesslich motorischer Einheiten), von Graefes Arch. Ophth., 152:731–744, 1952.

119. Reid, G., The rate of discharge of the extraocular motoneurones, J. Physiol., 110:217–225, 1949.

120. Sakatani, S., Ganka Rinsho I-ho, 49:409, 1955 (*cited by* Kuboki, 1957), and Ganka Rinsho I-ho, 49:803, 1955 (*cited by* Kuboki, 1957).

121. Sakatani, S., Electromyographic study in the ophthalmologic fields: Report IV, electromyographic study of normal and abnormal extraocular muscles regularity, Acta Soc. Ophth. Jap., 60:1080–1087, 1956.

122. Sears, M. L.; R. D. Teasdall; and H. H. Stone, Stretch effects in human extraocular muscle, an electromyographic study, Bull. Johns Hopk. Hosp., 104:174–178, 1959.

123. Serra, C., and A. Barone, Prime dati dell' esplorazione dell' attivita elettricca dei muscoli estrinsici oculari nella percezione di forma, Acta Neurol., 13:1010–1022, 1957.

124. Sherrington, C. S., Further experimental note on the correlation of action of antagonistic muscles, Proc. Roy. Soc., 53:407–420, 1893.

125. Sherrington, C. S., Experimental note on two movements of the eye, J. Physiol., 17:27–29, 1894.

126. Sherrington, C. S., Observations on the sensual role of the proprioceptive nerve supply of the extrinsic ocular muscles, Brain, 41:332–343, 1918.

127. Sherrington, C. S., The Integrative Action of the Nervous System. New Haven, Yale University Press, 1947.

128. Suzuki, S. (*cited by* Kuboki, Jap. J. Ophth., 3:66–74, 1959).

129. Tamler, E.; A. Jampolsky; and E. Marg, An electromyographic study of asymmetric convergence, Am. J. Ophth., 46:174–181, 1958.

130. Tamler, E.; E. Marg; and A. Jampolsky, An electromyographic study of coactivity of human extraocular muscles in following movements, A.M.A. Arch. Ophth., 61:270–273, 1959.

131. Tamler, E.; E. Marg; A. Jampolsky; and I. Nawratzki, Electromyography of human saccadic eye movements, A.M.A. Arch. Ophth., 62:657–661, 1959.

132. Tamler, E.; A. Jampolsky; and E. Marg, Electromyographic study of the following movements of the eye between tertiary positions, A.M.A. Arch. Ophth., 62:804–809, 1959.

133. Tamler, E.; A. Jampolsky; and E. Marg. Electromyography in strabismus, California Med., 90:437–439, 1959.

134. Tamler, E., Discussion of Tamler, Jampolsky, and Marg, 1958.

135. Tergast, P., Ueber des Verhältnis von Nerven und Muskel, Arch. Mikr. Anat., 9:36–46, 1873.

136. Thorson, J. C., and W. E. Bell, Progressive dystrophic external ophthalmoplegia with abiotrophic fundus changes, A.M.A. Arch. Ophth., 62:833–838, 1958.

137. Urist, M. J., Horizontal squint with secondary vertical deviations, A.M.A. Arch. Ophth., 46:245–267, 1951.

138. Van Allen, M. W., and F. C. Blodi, The Moebius syndrome, a case study with electromyography of the extraocular muscles, Am. J. Ophth. 45:926, 1958. (Abst.)

139. Walsh, F. B., Third nerve regeneration: A clinical evaluation, Brit. J. Ophth., 41:577–598, 1957.

140. Walton, J. N., The electromyogram in myopathy: Analysis with the audiofrequency spectrometer, J. Neurol. Neurosurg. & Psychiat., 15:219–226, 1952.

141. Weddell, G.; B. Feinstein; and R. E. Pattle, Electrical activity of voluntary muscle in man under normal and pathological conditions, Brain, 67:178–257, 1944.

142. Westheimer, G., Mechanism of saccadic eye movements, A.M.A. Arch. Ophth., 52:710–718, 1954.

143. Westheimer, G., and A. Mitchell, Eye movement responses to convergence stimuli, A.M.A. Arch. Ophth., 55:848–856, 1956.

144. Whitteridge, D., The effect of stimulation of intrafusal muscle fibers on sensitivity to stretch of extraocular muscle spindles, Quart. J. Exper. Physiol., 44:385–393, 1959.

145. York, F., and G. M. Breinin, Coding film recordings with the Grass Kymograph camera, Electroencephalog. & Clin. Neurophysiol. 11:362–364, 1959.

146. Van Allen, M.W., and F. C. Blodi, The effect of paralysis of the cervical sympathetic system on the electromyogram of extraocular muscles in the human, Am. J. Ophth. 49:679–683, 1960.

147. Rowley, P. T.; J. B. Wells; and R. L. Irwin, Tension response of mammalian muscle to intra-arterial acetylcholine, Am. J. Physiol., 198:507–510, 1960.

APPENDIX

NEEDLE ELECTRODES AS USED IN OCULAR ELECTROMYOGRAPHY

FREEMAN YORK, B.S.

Electrodes used in ocular electromyography consist of 27 to 31 gauge chrome steel hypodermic needles approximately 30 mm. in length through which is threaded a 44-gauge teflon-insulated copper wire. The larger gauge needles are used when skin penetration is called for, such as in inferior oblique recording, whereas the finer needles are inserted in the muscle directly through the conjunctiva.

Three basic types of electrodes are applicable for recording ocular electromyograms: (1) monopolar, solid steel or tungsten needles; (2) single coaxial (bipolar) needles, composed of one center conductor; (3) double or multiple coaxial needles, consisting of two or more center conductors inside a cannula. Monopolar needles can be made from ordinary insect pins of fine gauge (No. 000-1), which have first been stripped of their black paint, then sharpened to a tapered point, and reinsulated with varnish to the tip. They are used when it is desirable to record the electrical activity from a large area of muscle. Coaxial types, which are described fully below, are more suitable for clinical use. Fine-gauge coaxials have a limited pickup area and are often capable of resolving a few motor units. Double coaxials obviate grounding the patient by means of a separate wire since the cannula acts as the ground and the two inner conductors as the recording points; however, if one wishes, a patient ground wire may be used, in which the cannula would act as a shield ground.

The construction of coaxial electrodes involves many individual, sequential processes: first, the teflon-covered wire must be thoroughly insulated from the cannula with baking varnish. It is inserted through the cannula, dipped into varnish (that has been exposed to air for several minutes in order to become thickened), and drawn back and forth through the cannula several times, with dips into the varnish each time. When it can no longer be drawn easily, it is centered accurately, particularly at the tip end of the needle, and baked vertically in a constant-temperature oven at 150° F. for one to two hours. Higher temperatures will cause the varnish to bubble and break away from the steel.

After it has been baked, the teflon wire is cut off flush at the tip end and to about ½ inch of the handle end of the electrode. This ½-inch piece is then stripped of insulation for ¼ inch and silver-soldered to one lead of a twisted pair of 30-gauge nylon or plastic insulated hook-up wires. The other lead wire is stripped of insulation for ½ inch, tightly wrapped around the upper end of the cannula and also silver-soldered. Since chrome steel does not solder or weld well, a strong mechanical joint must be made; abrasing this joint area with carborundum and using 3 percent silver solder will help make a satisfactory electromechanical contact.

The exposed solder joints are then insulated with varnish and covered with a ¾-inch length of 18-gauge teflon or other suitable spaghetti tubing. Care must be taken that there is no electrical contact between the two soldered joints. This handle may also be made by molding epoxy resin or resistor cement around the upper end of the cannula and the ends of the lead wires. Sealing the ends of a teflon handle with epoxy resin will protect the joints and prevent the tube from sliding. Lead wires may be of fine-gauge, stranded wire (for flexibility), but their length should be kept to a minimum in order to reduce the electrical capacity and pickup of stray magnetic fields. They should also be color-coded, for it is sometimes necessary to change the polarity of the signal potential.

Insulating materials must meet rigid specifications as to chemical, electrical, and heat resistance. They must dry without excessive shrinking, hold up under attacks by sterilizing solutions, and be flexible enough to allow for slight electrode bending. Electrodes withstanding temperatures up to 105° C. are suitable for autoclaving, and insulators such as the epoxy resins, silicone-base laquers, baking varnishes, and teflon coverings will meet this requirement. Formvar-coated wire also can be used, but not types of wire with other enamels since they flake and are easily scratched. Voltage tolerance is not critical, as these electrodes, even when used for stimulating or coagulating purposes, carry minute amounts of current. Most varnishes are capable of taking several hundred volts at 100 percent relative humidity.

Pointing the tips of the electrodes is done with either a flat piece of No. 600 grit carborundum paper or a small hand motor tool having a carborundum wheel, rotating at slow speed. The tip may be a standard 60-degree bevel or a "pencil-point" type, and must be well polished and free from burrs. When polishing, no tiny particles of copper or steel can be allowed to become lodged between the center conductor and the cannula. With electrodes having more than one center conductor, it is especially critical that sufficient insulating material surround each wire, positioning it at an equal distance from other wires and from the cannula. A stereomicroscope with 40× magnification is helpful in this as well as in other construction steps.

Completed electrodes may be refined in two ways: by insulating the outside cannula, and by gold or silver plating. The latter technique is difficult and not essential for EMG recording; however, quieter traces and excellent base lines are obtained because of the reduction of D.C. potential between the electrode poles.

Commercial electroplating solutions are available, but the following formula of silver solution has worked best in this laboratory: 3.2 oz. per gal. silver cyanide, small amount of sodium carbonate, 4.5 oz. per gal. sodium cyanide, and 15 oz. per gal. potassium nitrate. Very low plating currents are used (the exact current depends, of course, on the area to be plated and the amount and concentration of silver in the solution). For needles under 1.5 inches long, 27 to 31 gauge less than 50 microamperes is needed for the center conductors and about 2 milliamperes for the barrel. The needle must be cleaned extremely well with carborundum and xylene; otherwise, gold or silver will flake off. With the electrode pole as the anode and a gold or silver bar in the solution as the cathode, the electrode is put into the solution and the current turned on slowly until small bubbles are seen rising from the electrode. A few seconds is usually all that is necessary for plating. Each pole is plated separately.

Chloriding electroplated electrodes with a chloride of the deposited element will further stabilize the pole pieces and render the electrode nonpolarizable. This is accomplished simply by placing the plated poles (each one separately) into the chloride bath and, using low voltage ratings (1 to 6 volts D.C.), reversing the electron flow two or three times, at intervals of 10 to 15 seconds. Gold and silver chloride require only very short duration, but platinum chloride takes almost twice as long to apply.

Insulation of the outside cannula is done in order to limit the surface area of conduction and also to reduce stray pickup. Viscous laquer, air-drying, or baking is used. An even layer must be applied from where the leads enter the handle down to the beveled tip of the cannula. This is accomplished by the use of a vertically mounted rack and pinion or similar fine-adjustment taxic device. The electrode is placed in this holder, dipped into a beaker of freshly-stirred laquer, and very slowly raised until the tip emerges. The bead of laquer that forms on the tip is carefully brushed off and the electrode is positioned tip upward and allowed to dry. After it has dried, the electrode tip is repolished, plated, if desired, and given a final test for insulation and conduction properties.

Resistance measurements are made throughout the construction procedure and any electrodes showing signs of insulation failure are immediately discarded. A megometer having an electrometer input and generating less than ten volts across the unknown resistance is used to check each coaxial electrode. The minimum resistance requirement for workable electrodes is approximately 50 to 100 megohms; however, values up to 10^{10} ohms are measurable in the heavier-gauge needles and are more acceptable for good recordings. Very-fine-gauge needles (No. 31) can have a measurement of between 10^6 and 10^8 ohms. Monopolar needles can be tested for insulation resistance by immersing them in a weak sodium chloride solution and passing 6 to 12 volts D.C. through them. Bubbling should appear only at the very tip of the electrode.

Impedance measurements may be made for individual electrodes by measuring their D.C. resistance in normal saline solution. Generally speaking, very-fine-gauge electrodes (No. 31) have high impedances, particularly double-coaxial 31 gauge (up to 100 Kohms), and one must make certain that one's recording amplifiers are able to handle such an input. Standard 29-gauge gold-plated coaxial electrodes have impedances of between 3.5 Kohms and 4.5 Kohms A.C. at 1000 cycles (measured with a Wheatstone bridge). D.C. measurements are about the same as A.C.

Sterilization of needle electrodes is usually carried out by immersing them in a noncorrosive solution such as zephiran chloride for at least fifteen minutes. Clinical use requires that only the barrel be sterilized, but for surgical procedures the entire assembly should be soaked or, if heat tolerances of the electrode elements permit, autoclaved.

Micro- and semimicroelectrodes of the metallic type can also be used for human extraocular muscle recording. Such electrodes may be fashioned from 70/30 percent platinum/iridium, stainless steel, or tungsten wires. The basic technique is as follows: (1) A solution of 50 percent sodium cyanide: 30 percent sodium hydroxide is made up as the bath used for electropolishing the wires. (2) Currents of about 1 amp, 12 to 15 volts A.C., are passed between the wire (positive) and the solution, initially for about 20 minutes, or until the wire has formed a blunt point of less than 100 microns as seen under a light microscope. Then the voltage is lowered to 1 to 6 volts A.C. for about the same period of time or until all bubbling ceases. If the voltage is graded finely enough, tip diameters of less than a micron can be obtained. (3) Insulation is applied, in the manner described above, except that, with microelectrodes, several coats of thinned laquer are applied with the electrode in an upright position. Because of the physical properties of such a small tip, several microns of height are almost always left exposed. (4) This insulated microelectrode must then be reinforced with a steel cannula by again coating it with varnish to the tip and inserting it into the barrel in much the same way as an ordinary coaxial electrode is made; however, the cannula tip is first beveled and the microelectrode tip drawn down until only the uninsulated part is exposed at the bevel. (5) Lead wires are attached. The electrode is not, of course, coated on the outside. Plating and chloriding may then be carried out.

Many methods for electrically reducing various types of wires exist and are described fully in the literature. Much individual experimenting has to be done, however, before one arrives at the right technique.

9 781442 652248